50 THINGS

YOU NEED TO KNOW ABOUT

DIABETES

Expert Tips for Taking Control

KATHLEEN STANLEY

CDE, CN, RD, LD, MSEd, BC-ADM

Director, Book Publishing, Robert Anthony; *Managing Editor, Book Publishing,* Abe Ogden; *Production Manager,* Melissa Sprott; *Cover Design,* Jody Billert; *Printer,* United Graphics Inc.

Printed in the United States of America
1 3 5 7 9 10 8 6 4 2

The suggestions and information contained in this publication are generally consistent with the *Clinical Practice Recommendations* and other policies of the American Diabetes Association, but they do not represent the policy or position of the Association or any of its boards or committees. Reasonable steps have been taken to ensure the accuracy of the information presented. However, the American Diabetes Association cannot ensure the safety or efficacy of any product or service described in this publication. Individuals are advised to consult a physician or other appropriate health care professional before undertaking any diet or exercise program or taking any medication referred to in this publication. Professionals must use and apply their own professional judgment, experience, and training and should not rely solely on the information contained in this publication before prescribing any diet, exercise, or medication. The American Diabetes Association—its officers, directors, employees, volunteers, and members—assumes no responsibility or liability for personal or other injury, loss, or damage that may result from the suggestions or information in this publication.

⊗ The paper in this publication meets the requirements of the ANSI Standard Z39.48-1992 (permanence of paper).

ADA titles may be purchased for business or promotional use or for special sales. To purchase more than 50 copies of this book at a discount, or for custom editions of this book with your logo, contact the American Diabetes Association at the address below, at booksales@diabetes.org, or by calling 703-299-2046.

American Diabetes Association
1701 North Beauregard Street
Alexandria, Virginia 22311

Library of Congress Cataloging-in-Publication Data

Stanley, Kathleen, 1963-
50 things you need to know about your diabetes care--right now! / by Kathleen Stanley.
    p. cm.
Includes bibliographical references and index.
ISBN 978-1-58040-283-5 (alk. paper)
1. Diabetes--Popular works. I. Title. II. Title: Fifty things you need to know about your diabetes care--right now!
RC660.4.S73 2009
616.4'62--dc22

2009005564

To George, Alex, and Steve with love.

*Thanks to my furry, supportive companions,
Coco (now departed) and Frankie,
who kept me company many late hours
to complete this project.*

CONTENTS

CHAPTER 5. DO YOUR DAILY ACTIVITIES

CHAPTER 6. WHAT ELSE CAN AFFECT YOUR BLOOD GLUCOSE?

CHAPTER 7. DEAL WITH SPECIAL HEALTH ISSUES

CHAPTER 8. PREVENT PROBLEMS DOWN THE ROAD

CHAPTER 9. DEAL WITH SOME UNEXPECTED PROBLEMS

CHAPTER 10. AVOID FEELING "LABELED"

PREFACE

As diabetes care has advanced over the years with new gadgets, tools, and methods, one principle has remained the same: Education is the key to successful diabetes self-care and optimal health. The new, little bright-colored meters are cool, and insulin delivery devices (pumps and pods) are sophisticated, but if you don't know how to solve problems for yourself, these tools can only help so much.

Diabetes education can come from formal training with a health care professional—a physician, certified diabetes educator (CDE), nurse, registered dietitian (RD), or pharmacist—and from informal experiences in life. Qualified health care professionals can teach basic self-care strategies and provide useful information. But real life situations, such as eating out at a restaurant for the first time after being diagnosed, will test your ability to apply your knowledge to different settings and situations. There are challenges to face daily, and some are easier to conquer than others.

The goal of this book is to help make a link between the skills you learn from health care professionals and the real-life situations you will face. The

> "The goal of this book is to help make a link between the skills you learn from health care professionals and the real-life situations you will face."

intent of the book is not to replace diabetes education classes, as you need to have a basic understanding of diabetes and a basic set of skills. Learning how to test your blood glucose, develop a meal plan, or take medications are best learned in a formal setting with hands-on instruction. But your body will also teach you how it works and responds to situations, which may vary slightly from the theory you learned in class, or even in this book. You will need to develop your own unique strategies and solutions for certain circumstances along the way at times.

Diabetes care is constantly evolving and improving. New products are developed each year that can directly improve your quality of life, and you will want to be in the know about these new products. You will also learn to modify your own management strategies when an outcome wasn't what you expected or planned for. Sometimes in diabetes, you have to make an educated guess to predict what will happen to your blood glucose in a situation. Your personal blood glucose monitor device is an indispensable tool to use to help you collect information about outcomes and learn from past unexpected situations to face the new ones.

Finally, be open to making changes in your own care as you live with diabetes. Your body will go through natural changes each year, and these changes will require adjustments on your part. Use resources, such as your personal health care team and information from the American Diabetes Association (ADA), to help you make informed decisions about your health. Share any successful tips you have learned with others who live with diabetes, too. Imparting strategies and ideas you have learned to others can help you build a support network and improve your own knowledge. Isn't it often said that teachers learn more from their students than the other way around?

The truth is that you will be a lifelong student in the subject of diabetes. But it will be a journey that is worthwhile. My hope is that this book can help. In the following pages, I provide useful tips derived from professional experts, as well as "real life" people. The result is the first "50 Things" you should know about diabetes.

—*Kathleen Stanley, CDE, RD, LD, CN, MSEd, BC-ADM*

CHAPTER 1
KNOW THE PLAYERS

---

1. How to pick a good diabetes doctor and get the most out of the relationship

---

2. How to interpret an A1C score

---

3. How to get the most out of your visit to the registered dietitian

---

4. How to call your doctor for help

---

5. How to work with your insurance company

How to pick a good diabetes doctor and get the most out of the relationship

FINDING YOUR DOCTOR

Diabetes is a lifelong disease, so choosing a good doctor to take care of your diabetes will be a long-term decision. Think about other relationships you have established for your business or in your personal life. More than likely, good communication and trust are largely responsible for the successful relationships you have had. You will be working together with a doctor for years, so choose carefully, and expect to build the relationship over time, not just at the first visit. The following tips should help you in this important search.

GET PROFESSIONAL ADVICE

Ask your favorite current health care provider (family doctor, dentist, ophthalmologist) to recommend someone. If you like this provider's professional style, chances are, they will recommend someone who uses a similar style.

DO SOME SCOUTING BEFOREHAND

Some physician offices and clinics have marketing packets or office information packets that could be mailed to you. The web is also an excellent resource. Many insurance companies, hospitals, and even municipal websites offer online physician finders. Many doctors and clinics also have their own website with information on credentials, services, and insurance policies.

CONSIDER COMMUNICATION STYLES

Start your selection process by considering your communication needs and preferences. If you are the type who likes to have frequent contact or ask a lot of questions, you might want to consider a physician who has an on-call resource for after hours or enough trained staff to answer questions when the physician isn't available. Ask if the health care professional or physician takes direct calls, or if you are routed to others or through a frustrating electronic messaging center ("press 1 for more options, press 2 if you are tired of options, press 3 if you want us to disconnect you for no apparent reason, press 4 if you would like to throw your phone across the room"). If you are very comfortable with technology, seek out a doctor who is using the latest technology in their office (see sidebar).

HOW MUCH TIME DO YOU NEED?

If you prefer one-on-one time with a human being, you may want to ask about the time slots for appointments, or even take a casual visit to see the waiting room. If appointments are scheduled every 10 minutes, the waiting room is overflowing, and the staff looks harried, it may be sign that you may not get a lot of face-to-face time with this particular doctor. Conversely, some offices employ support

Making Peace with Diabetes Technology

Many of us could happily live our lives without owning an MP3 player or sending a text message. But when it comes to your diabetes care, it's time to accept some degree of technology, because it will to play an ever more important role in your health. For instance, some physicians use health data banks and software that allow you to input your blood glucose information and management information online. You can send in your numbers and get an update on your management without setting foot into a doctor's office! Many health care professionals also communicate through e-mail, which can sometimes be more reliable than a phone call. And let's not forget the number of diabetes management software programs available on cell phones, personal organizers, and computers. Most of these are very easy to learn and can make organizing data, analyzing your numbers, and spotting trends much, much easier.

So even if you wouldn't own a digital camera if someone paid you, it might be time to accept that some technology can simplify your diabetes management and improve your health.

persons to help with your visit, including a dietitian, laboratory staff, and diabetes educators. With this extra staff, you will probably get more personal contact. You will also get the scheduling flexibility of a multidisciplinary team, rather than being dependent on just one person. Remember that diabetes is a multifaceted problem, and a team can help in your overall health care treatment plan.

GROUP PRACTICES VERSUS SOLO PRACTITIONERS

Larger offices may have several partners, so ask if you will (or can) be assigned to one particular physician, allowing you to develop a relationship if that is important to you. If not, you may be scheduled with the "available" physician when you call, meaning you may be seeing a number of physicians or professionals. Finding someone you "click" with and can talk openly with is very important; you are developing relationships that will undoubtedly grow over the years.

CHECK THEM OUT AT A CHECKUP

The best time to make the first visit is for a simple checkup. This way you can see how the office works and meet the physician without the stress of an illness. At each visit you should generally expect:

- ▋ Weight check
- ▋ Blood pressure check
- ▋ Physical exam
- ▋ Feet and leg check (skin, circulation, and feeling)
- ▋ Current medication review (take vials and bottles so they can verify them)
- ▋ Home management plan review (diet, activity, and medications)
- ▋ Blood glucose log book or records review (looking for highs, lows, and trends)
- ▋ Lab work
- ▋ Time for questions and answers
- ▋ Discussion on preventative measures
- ▋ A plan for your care
- ▋ An appointment time for your next visit

After the visit, consider how it went. If the checkup wasn't thorough or the conversations didn't go well, this may not be a good sign for when you have an urgent need or problem in the future.

NEIGHBORLY ADVICE

When choosing a doctor, common sense has you looking to neighbors and friends for a recommendation. This is indeed a good idea, as long as you also keep in mind that a friendly personality does not always mean quality care. When you get a recommendation, follow up by asking your neighbors and friends to describe their diabetes control. They might have a nice, friendly doctor, but if that physician is allowing your neighbor to have a long-term A1C higher than 8% or continuous unsolved glucose swings, well, it should raise some red flags.

PICK THE BEST

Fortunately, there are established standards of care that exist for diabetes management published by the American Diabetes Association (ADA). You may want to get to know these standards by visiting the ADA website (www.diabetes.org), calling the toll-free number (1-800-DIABETES), or asking a certified diabetes educator

---

FINDING PHYSICIANS ONLINE

To find an endocrinologist in your area, try the following websites, which have physician search options.

Web Address	Site Sponsor
www.ncqa.org	National Committee for Quality Assurance
www.diabetes.org	American Diabetes Association
www.dlife.com	dlife Incorporated
www.aace.com	American Association of Clinical Endocrinologists
www.ama-assn.org	American Medical Association
www.healthfinder.gov	U.S. Department of Health and Human Services
www.abms.org	American Board of Medical Specialists

Many insurance providers have online physician finders that also list affiliations and accreditations. These finders offer the benefit of looking specifically for doctors that accept your insurance. Finally, your state medical association should also have information online.

(CDE). Physicians who have met these established national standards can apply for a unique voluntary status known as "American Diabetes Association Recognized Provider." This rigorous application signifies that the physician has achieved and maintained national standards of care in diabetes. Something else to note—this is a volunteer process that takes time and effort. The mere fact that the physician felt it important enough to pursue can say a lot. To find a physician who has achieved this recognition, go to http://recognition.ncqa.org.

INVESTIGATE THE RECORDS

Find out what your potential provider's qualifications are and how long they have had them. The local state medical board may be able to provide you with information about physician status and previous outcomes. In the near future, doctors may also have "report cards" available on the Internet that will provide you with information about quality of care. In addition to the physician, do your homework on the other staff members. Some offices use physician assistants or nurse practitioners to help with the growing numbers of patients. These health care professionals also have state licensing boards that can be contacted for researching information.

WHERE WILL THEY SEND YOU?

Consider the hospital or diagnostic centers your potential physician is affiliated with. If you are not impressed with the facilities to which they will refer you, it could add undue stress when a need or emergency arises. Check to see if the center or facility has a CDE on staff (search for individual CDEs at www.aade.net), or has achieved American Diabetes Association Recognition (search for recognized sites at www.diabetes.org). Also ask where you will receive diabetes education classes—a pamphlet on "diet" and a free meter won't do.

LOCATION, LOCATION, LOCATION

This may seem like an unimportant detail, but the location of your doctor's office can affect how willing you are to make appointments. You will more than likely require several checkups or "well visits" during the year, so carefully evaluate the location of the physician (including their parking areas!). Make sure you have reliable and accessible transportation to the office. If you have a good relationship with your doctor, it may be worth a longer trip. However, don't set yourself up for a long drive if you feel it will keep you from making regular appointments. Missing check-up appointments will disrupt your physician's ability to perform preventative assessments and interventions for your future health.

ONCE YOU'VE DECIDED ON A DOCTOR

BE CONSIDERATE

Remember the doctor-patient relationship is a two-way street. No-show appointments are a pain for physician offices, as they are lost time that could have been made available to another person in need. Be considerate. If you make an appointment, stick with it, or call well in advance to reschedule. When calling, talk with the staff with the understanding that you are not the only patient in the practice, and that some demands may take longer than what you anticipated. Staff remember bad-tempered patients as well as patients remember bad-tempered staff.

MAKE THE MOST OF YOUR VISIT

Bring the following items to your appointment. Doing so can mean a more efficient and thorough visit for you and your health care providers.

- Specific list of questions and concerns (don't leave it up to the doctor to ask all the right questions, or expect him or her to be a mind reader)
- Blood glucose meter for downloading
- Accurate (and honest) blood glucose diary (hand written or computer-generated)
- Easy to remove footwear—to allow a foot inspection (if your doctor doesn't do this at each visit, make them)
- List of current medications, including over-the-counter products and nutritional supplements
- An update on recent illnesses or ongoing health problems (be sure to fill out that sometimes-lengthy health

questionnaire at your visits and update it when changes occur, even though it is tedious)

∎ Current insurance card(s)
∎ Name and phone number of current pharmacy to refill or renew prescriptions (will save you both a phone call later)
∎ Paper and pen for writing down new information or instructions
∎ A friend or family member who can help provide both support and a second set of ears to hear and remember the information provided during the visit

If you leave the appointment feeling you need more time and assistance understanding diabetes care, ask to be referred to a diabetes education class. Use available resources such as diabetes-related magazines, books, cookbooks, websites, and local support groups. Call your local ADA office to find out about these and other hometown and national resources.

MORE RESOURCES TO EXPLORE

MAGAZINES, JOURNALS, AND OTHER PERIODICALS

Position statement: Standards of medical care in diabetes. American Diabetes Association. *Diabetes Care* 30:S4–41, 2007

BOOKS

Diabetes Type 2 and What to Do, 2nd edition, by Virginia Valentine, June Biermann, and Barbara Toohey. Lowell House; Los Angeles, CA. 1998.

YOU—The Smart Patient: An Insider's Handbook for Getting the Best Treatment, by Michael F. Rozen and Mehmet C. Oz, with The Joint Commission. Free Press; New York, NY. 2006.

WEBSITES

American Diabetes Association . . . . WWW.DIABETES.ORG

National Committee for Quality Assurance . . WWW.NCQA.ORG

(continued)

WEBSITES *(continued)*

dlife Incorporated . . . . WWW.DLIFE.COM

American Association of Clinical
  Endocrinologists . . . . WWW.AACE.COM

American Medical Association . . . . WWW.AMA-ASSN.ORG

U.S. Department of Health and
  Human Services . . . . WWW.HEALTHFINDER.GOV

American Board of Medical Specialists . . . . . WWW.ABMS.ORG

2

How to interpret an A1C score

THE FACTS ARE IN

Since 1987, research has proven that blood glucose numbers are directly related to future diabetes complications. The landmark Diabetes Control and Complications Trial (DCCT) provided clear evidence that poor glucose control increases the risk of certain types of diabetes complications, including eye, kidney, and nerve damage in those with type 1 diabetes. Other studies followed individuals with type 2 diabetes and demonstrated that lowering average blood glucose could reduce similar complications. For both forms of diabetes, better blood glucose control over time means less chance of complications.

"Better blood glucose control over time means less chance of complications."

Blood glucose numbers change minute by minute. There are 1440 minutes in a day, so if you want a continuous snapshot of your blood glucose, you're in for a lot of finger pricks (or a continuous glucose monitor, which we'll discuss later). Fortunately, there is a test that will show you what your average blood glucose levels have been over a 3-month period of time. The Hemoglobin A1$_C$ (A1C) test is a blood test that measures what your average blood glucose has been for the last 90–120 days. Some other names you may hear or see for this type of test are "glycohemoglobin," "HbA1c," or simply "your percentage." The preferred reference is "A1C." This number is an important figure in your diabetes control game plan. Single glucose checks are important, but they can sometimes be misleading. Nothing gives you a better understanding of your overall diabetes control than your A1C.

WHAT IS AN A1C TEST?

A1C is short for a type of hemoglobin, which is a protein found inside your red blood cells. Hemoglobin performs several essential functions, such as carrying oxygen to the cells in your body. It also carries glucose. An A1C check looks at the amount of this glucose to determine your average blood glucose.

To understand how this test works, imagine your arteries and veins as structures forming highways though which liquids and solids can travel. Now imagine that your blood is the traffic on these highways. Blood isn't just a uniform liquid—it contains a variety of types of cells within its liquid mass, and red blood cells are one of the cell types present. As blood moves throughout your body, the glucose that is also present in the liquid highway will stick to the red blood cell. In other words, it binds, or "glyco-sylates" with the blood cell's hemoglobin. The more glucose that is in the blood, the more glucose will be found sticking to the hemoglobin. Since the red blood cell lives about 90 days, an A1C test involves looking at mature red blood cells and seeing how much glucose is found sticking to them. The amount is measured in terms of a percentage. For example, an A1C result of 6% means that 6% of the hemoglobin tested has glucose stuck to it.

Keep in mind that there are some circumstances that can affect the accuracy of an A1C result. If you have recently had a blood transfusion, suffered significant blood loss, or you suffer from some forms of anemia you should discuss your condition with your health care provider.

WHAT IS NORMAL?

Depending on the laboratory your physician uses, the normal range of an A1C level is about 4–6%. Check with your physician about what reference range is used, as it is normal to see some variation between laboratory reports, depending on how the analysis is performed. A 4–6% A1C level compares to an average blood glucose level of approximately 70–120 mg/dl, which is considered to be "normal."

The American Diabetes Association recommends people with diabetes keep their A1C levels below 7% (lower for some), which is a glucose reading of approximately 150 mg/dl on average over a 2–3 month period. (The American Association of Clinical Endocrinologists supports a slightly lower goal of less than 6.5%, equal to about 140 mg/dl over the same period of time.) Discuss your own target with your health care team. There may be times when your target might need to change (during pregnancy, when treated for other health problems, etc.).

THE WORD "AVERAGE" IS KEY

While an A1C check provides great information, it is not a replacement for daily blood glucose testing. Your daily tests should be reviewed alongside an A1C test to help you understand your daily and overall control. Because A1C is an average, it will not show if you are having problems with hypoglycemia or experiencing unstable readings. It is an important test, but trends in your daily blood glucose cannot be identified by A1C results alone.

WHERE DO YOU HAVE AN A1C CHECK DONE?

A1C checks are usually done at your doctor's office, either with equipment on the premises or through a blood sample that is drawn and sent to a laboratory. The result will be sent to the office in a few days to a week. Make sure you get the result and discuss it with your health care providers.

HOW OFTEN SHOULD AN A1C CHECK BE DONE?

The American Diabetes Association currently recommends you have an A1C done twice a year if you are meeting treatment goals and quarterly (every 3 months) if your therapy has changed, or you're not meeting treatment goals. An A1C will not generally be repeated any sooner than 2 months from the last check unless special circumstances warrant it.

ESTIMATED AVERAGE GLUCOSE

The term estimated average glucose, or eAG for short, is a new way of showing average blood glucose information in the same units (mg/dl) that people are used to seeing on their meters and glucose lab reports, rather than using a percentage like A1C. A1C percentage is sometimes confusing to people, so having your results in terms of a meter value may make the information more realistic and intriguing. Still, it's simply a different way of showing the same thing—your average glucose over a period of months.

IS YOUR A1C THE SAME AS YOUR eAG?

Not exactly, but it is another way to interpret your control. The eAG will soon be the standard reporting value for health care providers and patients, so you should know how the two values relate to one another. The following is a chart that shows how the two results compare:

A1C %	eAG mg/dl	A1C %	eAG mg/dl	A1C %	eAG mg/dl
6	126 mg/dl	7.5	169 mg/dl	9	212 mg/dl
6.5	140 mg/dl	8	183 mg/dl	9.5	226 mg/dl
7	154 mg/dl	8.5	197 mg/dl	10	240 mg/dl

IS THE "AVERAGE" REPORTED ON YOUR BLOOD GLUCOSE METER THE SAME AS eAG?

No. The "average" on your meter only reflects the average from the readings you performed. If you only check a few times a day like most people, you only have a few points of data, and not the constant data that's represented by an eAG or A1C check. The eAG reflects what your blood glucose readings were 24/7 for 3 months.

ONCE YOU HAVE YOUR RESULT

YOUR A1C IS HIGHER THAN 7%. WHAT NOW?

If your test result is higher than your target, immediately discuss with your health care providers what you can do to improve your results in the future. Don't wait until the next visit! Consider your management plan and ask yourself:

HOW DO YOU CALCULATE YOUR eAG?

You can calculate your eAG using your current A1C result. The formula is as follows:

$$(28.7 \times A1C) - 46.7 = eAG$$

It's probably been a while since math class, so an example to illustrate may make it more clear. Let's say your A1C is 8.2%. For the formula, you treat your A1C result simply as a number and not a percentage. So to calculate your eAG, you would first multiply 28.7 by 8.2 (your A1C):

$$28.7 \times 8.2 = 235.34$$

Now, you would take this number, 235.34, and subtract 46.7:

$$235.34 - 46.7 = 188.64$$

Then just round up to the nearest whole number, 189, and you have your eAG. In this case, that would be an average blood glucose of 189 mg/dl over a 3-month period. Seeing this should illustrate how eAG is useful. If your doctor says you have an A1C of 8.2%, you probably realize that is high, but it can also be just another number. However, if your doctor says your blood glucose level averages 189 mg/dl, you have a much more concrete idea of what that means. Mostly, it means you've got some work to do!

▌ Is your nutrition plan working out?
▌ Are you consistent with your activity plan?
▌ Are you following prescribed medication schedules?
▌ Are there other factors contributing to your control (for example, stress, other health problems, other medications, chronic pain)?

Learn what options your health care providers have to suggest. A high A1C is not simply your fault; it is a problem to be dealt with by you and your health care team.

> A high A1C is not simply your fault.

WHAT IF YOUR SELF GLUCOSE CHECKS DON'T MATCH YOUR A1C?

It is possible your blood glucose meter may need to be replaced, or you're not following the manufacturer's guidelines. However, it's more likely that the variation comes from the different nature of each test. An A1C only reports an average—it cannot show daily fluctuations. Conversely, you may need to do your self glucose checks at different times of the day. Always checking at the same times of day will limit your ability to fully understand your glucose levels over a 24-hour period.

Remember, an A1C result of 7% compares to a blood glucose average of about 150 mg/dl. Think of how many different ways you can mathematically achieve this average, even with just two blood glucose numbers obtained each day during a month. Consider the individuals below:

Person with A1C of 7%	Actual home glucose results
Joe	100 mg/dl and 200 mg/dl
Jane	75 mg/dl and 225 mg/dl
Jill	50 mg/dl and 250 mg/dl
John	140 mg/dl and 160 mg/dl

WILL CONTINUOUS GLUCOSE MONITORING REPLACE A1C?

Continuous glucose monitoring (CGM) appears to be the future of self blood glucose testing. By using a device that continually checks blood glucose levels, these systems provide a complete view of levels throughout the day, improving glucose management and overall self-care. However, CGM devices aren't perfect yet and many are expensive or hard to get; more work certainly needs to be done. Whether they will replace A1C tests remains to be seen, but it's hard to imagine that an overall glucose snapshot of a 2–3 month period won't be useful in the future. Likely, CGM will be an excellent tool to use alongside an A1C check. For now, all individuals with diabetes, whether they use a meter, or CGM devices, should have an A1C check to be evaluated alongside daily readings, whether from a meter or a properly calibrated CGM device.

All four of these individuals have the same A1C, yet their control is obviously not the same. Jill and Jane are experiencing big, out-of-control swings, and Joe and John are not consistently in the 70–140 mg/dl range. Having this type of information can put your A1C results into perspective.

DO YOU STILL NEED TO KEEP A BLOOD GLUCOSE LOG BOOK?

There's no replacement for a well-kept glucose log book. Always take your logbook (or a meter with a memory function) to appointments. Ask every member of your health care team to review the information, including your educator, nurse, pharmacist, or dietitian. Compare your logbook results with the A1C results on a daily, weekly, or monthly basis and not just every 2–3 months.

MORE RESOURCES TO EXPLORE

BOOKS

Diabetes A to Z: What You Need to Know About Diabetes—Simply Put, 5th edition. American Diabetes Association; Alexandria, VA, 2003.

WEBSITES

American Diabetes Association Website . . . . WWW.DIABETES.ORG

How to get the most out of your visit to the registered dietitian

Visiting a registered dietitian (RD) seems to be as popular as going to the dentist to have a cavity filled. Maybe less so. Perhaps people cringe at the thought of exposing their personal food choices and body weight to a RD. Perhaps they expect to be scolded or judged. Unfortunately, many physicians have not exactly helped put these perceptions to rest. In some cases, the physician may even use the threat of an appointment with a RD as some strange motivational tactic to encourage patients to change behaviors. Not surprisingly, this tactic doesn't work, but it does turn the RD into the boogeyman. In other cases, health care professionals will make offhand, negative comments such as, "You won't be able to eat THAT anymore," and then set up an appointment without a patient's consent, creating a scenario where the individual anticipates having things taken away from them before they even step through the door.

Here's the good news about a referral to a RD—it is not punishment, it is valuable. The RD is a vital member of your diabetes health care team and a terrific source of nutrition information. In fact, most people find that a RD expands their food choices as opposed to limiting them. Considering the other options for nutrition education—food advice from a copied menu or an article from a popular magazine—it's not surprising that most enjoy the special attention and conversation

WHAT'S A RD?

Once you realize a RD is not a dietary dictator or the food police, you might wonder what a RD actually is. Following are some characteristics all RDs share.

- RDs are food and nutrition experts.
- RDs have attained at least a Bachelor's Degree.
- RDs have completed coursework and supervised practice accredited by the Commission on Accreditation for Dietetic Education (CADE).
- RDs have had to pass a national exam by the Commission on Dietetic Registration (CDR).
- RDs must continue their training by achieving a certain number of educational requirements each year (in other words, they must stay up to date).
- RDs work in hospitals, clinics, health care facilities, wellness programs, food industries, private practices, public health services, universities, research facilities, culinary institutions, schools, cooperative extension services, and government agencies.
- RDs in diabetes care follow precise practice guidelines, to assure quality.
- RDs come in all shapes, ages, and sizes, and either gender; they are human, after all.
- RDs want to help you, not punish you.

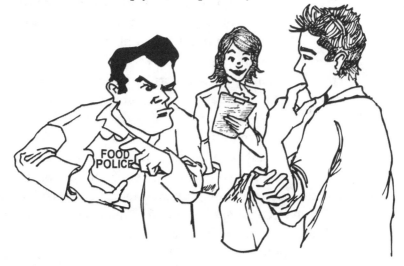

DOES A RD VISIT COST MONEY?

A visit to the RD will likely mean an out-of-pocket cost. Find out from your insurance company in advance what will be covered and what will not be covered. Medicare does provide coverage for meeting with RDs under certain conditions, and many private insurance policies will cover appointments if the RD is associated with an American Diabetes Association Recognized Diabetes Education Program or American Association of Diabetes Educator's Accredited Program (see the box How to Find a Professional). With so much "free" nutrition information out on the web, on newsstands, and in magazine racks (some of it valid, most of it utter nonsense), many people wonder why they should pay a RD. It helps to remember they are medically and professionally trained and they are working with you. There is a lot of free general medical advice available as well, but we still understand the importance of visiting our doctor for a checkup. The same is true of a RD.

WHAT WILL YOU GET FROM YOUR VISIT?

Meeting a RD is much more personal and useful than being given a free "diet sheet" from a tear pad at the doctor's office. Why? Because you are an individual. From the minute you started putting food in your mouth, your reaction to food was unique. At about 12–18 months old, when you became independent with your spoon, you gained control of what you did and did not put in your mouth. From that time on, you learned to make your own choices.

> You are an individual. From the minute you started putting food in your mouth, your reaction to food was unique.

An individualized plan designed for people with diabetes allows choices as well. How could a copy of a preprinted 1800-calorie diet with a one-day menu possibly work for everyone? People with diabetes come in different ages, sizes, and shapes and each has different medical needs. One plan does not fit all. To make sure you get the most of your appointment, ideally ask for a consultation with an established American Diabetes Association Recognized Program or American Association of Diabetes Educator's Accredited Program. Look for someone who is a Certified Diabetes Educator (CDE). A CDE is a professional who

HOW TO FIND A PROFESSIONAL

What you are looking for	Where to find it
Registered Dietitian	www.eatright.org
The American Dietetic Association is the largest dietitian organization in the U.S., and is considered an authority on nutrition information in the U.S.	1-800-877-1600
Recognized Education Program	www.diabetes.org
The American Diabetes Association provides a full listing of all Recognized Education Programs. The programs must meet a variety of standards.	1-800-DIABETES
Certified Diabetes Educator	www.diabeteseducator.org
The American Association of Diabetes Educators is the nation's largest association of diabetes educators. They also provide accreditation to education programs based on standards.	1-800-338-3633

has met standards and passed a qualified exam to be designated as someone knowledgeable and experienced in diabetes care. See the box How to Find a Professional for more information on how to find these professionals.

GET THE MOST OUT OF YOUR VISIT TO THE RD

ASK YOURSELF WHAT YOU WANT OUT OF THE VISIT

Do some soul-searching before your appointment and determine what you want to learn from your visit. You will also likely be asked to make some changes; what are you willing to do? You should be in a state of mind to receive suggestions and act on them. If you feel your first RD doesn't meet your needs, don't give up; ask for another RD.

STAY POSITIVE

Forget the negatives you've heard in the past and start from scratch. If you are anticipating the worst, this negativity will set the stage and will become the inevitable outcome of the visit. Unfortunately, friends, family members, and health care professionals may have said some unkind and hurtful things to you about your weight, food choices, or food behaviors. Start your new relationship by viewing the RD as someone who is there to support you, and remember that it may take a few visits to formulate the right plan.

BE TRUTHFUL

Hiding information about your eating habits or behaviors will make it impossible to develop a personalized meal plan that can work. For instance, if you have a weekly date out with friends at a local restaurant, tell the RD. He or she can help you make the best choices at this restaurant and not force you to give up important parts of your lifestyle. Tell the RD what your favorite foods are—any plan that cuts out these foods completely will be difficult to follow.

SET SHORT-TERM AND LONG-TERM GOALS

Goal planning is an essential part of changing habits. Food habits have taken years to establish and will take time to change. A proper goal should answer three questions:

1. What? What you want to achieve (the change)
2. When? When you plan to achieve it (the timeline)
3. How? How you will achieve it (the strategy)

EXAMPLE: *"I will substitute a 15-gram carbohydrate food choice for my mid-morning snack at work instead of a candy bar (1). I will start doing this next Monday (2). I will go to the store on Saturday and select some new things that have about 15 grams of carbohydrate in them (3)."*

> Whatever you do, do not call your meal plan a diet.

Without these three elements, it is difficult to initiate change. During your appointment, write down your goal and include these elements to provide a clear concept of your plan. Your goals should be realistic—losing 20 pounds overnight is not a good short-term goal. In setting only a few realistic goals at a time, you will be better able to make changes that will last a lifetime, rather than just a few days.

REMEMBER, NO ONE'S PERFECT

No matter how great your meal plan, there are going to be times when you fall off the wagon. Ask your RD about relapse prevention and strategies on what to do if you get off track. One very important tip: Do not call your plan a "diet." This word has a negative and short-term implication. Medical literature calls it a "medical nutrition plan," but most RDs will simply call it a meal or nutrition plan. Another word to drop from your food vocabulary: "cheating." Instead, you make "choices" with food. Learning how to incorporate your favorite foods into your plan will help you stick with your plan.

BRING IN A FOOD DIARY

A food diary can help you identify some previously unrecognized food behaviors, such as unconscious eating (nibbling while you cook, snacking while watching TV, grabbing a handful of something as you breeze through the kitchen) or nervous snacking (eating while you are stressed or nervous). See the food diary sample in Table 1 for an example.

TABLE 1. SAMPLE FOOD DIARY

Food	Amount	Time	Place	Reason for Eating (hungry/ nervous/ don't know)	Others present	Did it satisfy?	Other notes

TAKE THE SHOPPER AND CHEF WITH YOU

The person who prepares your food should, if possible, accompany you to the RD visit. No, this does not mean you should hunt down Ronald McDonald. But if your wife or husband does the cooking for you, they should learn what you learn. Knowing what to buy and how to prepare the food is an important part of putting together the pieces of a meal plan. Ultimately, though, *the responsibility to follow the plan falls on the person who holds the fork.*

TAKE MENUS AND EMPTY BOXES WITH YOU

If you visit a particular restaurant on a regular basis, ask for a menu and bring it with you to your RD visit. With this information, you and the RD can identify healthy choices and develop strategies for eating healthier while eating out. The same is true for some of your favorite boxed foods—take in the label. With your real-life tools (menus, labels, etc.), you will be able to individualize your plan and practice making choices.

COMPLETE A NUTRITIONAL ASSESSMENT

Ideally, your RD will have you to complete a nutritional assessment, which should ask for:

- Food likes and dislikes
- Food allergy history
- Current weight
- Past weight
- Current health status and medications
- Food intolerances
- Swallowing abilities
- Digestive problems
- Food purchasing needs
- Food preparation styles
- Restaurant dining habits
- Alcohol use

ASK FOR A FOLLOW-UP

Determine when the next visit will be, or how a follow-up will be handled after your visit. A follow-up will give you the opportunity to discuss real-life experiences you've encountered with your meal plan, what things work, and what may need some more planning. The RD can provide a source of support and encouragement for whatever your goals are, so use your resources and stay in touch. Once you've established a meal plan, it may help to touch base with your RD annually to discuss new food choices and any new information that may help you improve your plan.

MORE RESOURCES TO EXPLORE

WEBSITES

American Diabetes Association Website . . . . WWW.DIABETES.ORG

American Dietetic Association . . . . WWW.EATRIGHT.ORG

American Association of
  Diabetes Educators . . . . WWW.DIABETESEDUCATOR.ORG

4

How to call your doctor for help

There will be days with unexpected troubles, days when you need to get some advice from your health care team about your diabetes care. The doctor's office is the place for getting accurate medical advice. It may be easier to ask friends or neighbors (or the Internet) for health advice, but they may unknowingly provide you with misinformation, or worse yet, provide dangerous suggestions, which could cause further problems. Here is some good advice for when you need some help.

DISCUSS THE GROUND RULES

Ideally, as part of your initial visit, you should have been given information from your health care team about when to contact them, your responsibilities when doing so, and when interventions are up to them. If you have not received this information, plan to ask these questions at your next visit:

- At what levels do you want me to treat high or low blood glucose on my own?
- What number should I call when my blood glucose gets really high (for example, higher than 350 mg/dl)?
- What number should I call for help when my blood glucose gets really low (for example, lower than 50 mg/dl)?
- When should I call other health care professionals instead of you?
- Should I call you if I experience any hypoglycemia, or just moderate to severe episodes?
- Should I have a glucagon emergency kit?

- Should I check for ketones? If yes, when?
- What steps should I take if I have positive ketones?
- What steps should I take if I can't take my diabetes medication (going to have a dental procedure, employment physical, having vomiting, etc.)?
- What steps should I take if I run out of medication?
- What steps should I take if I can't reach your office for a diabetes problem?
- Who will be taking my after-hour calls? What are his or her professional qualifications? Do they have access to my medical history if needed?
- When should I go to the hospital if I can't manage my blood glucoses on my own?
- To which hospital should I go if I need emergency help?

WHEN TO CALL

Typically, you will want to notify your health care provider at once if:

- You run out of medication
- You are running a fever (for more than 8 hours)
- You are unable to eat (nausea, vomiting, diarrhea, other) for more than 6 hours
- You have missed more than one dose of diabetes medication
- You are spilling moderate (or greater) ketones, or cannot clear trace/small ketones
- You have symptoms of diabetic ketoacidosis (DKA) if you have type 1 diabetes
- You are having "runaway" high blood glucose levels for a few hours (starting at 200, then moving up to 300, then going to 400. Do I hear 450?)

EMERGENCY SITUATIONS—TAKE ACTION

If you are experiencing symptoms of a serious health problem, such as a serious injury, possible heart attack or stroke, or possible DKA, do not call your doctor's office. Have someone take you to the nearest hospital or call your local emergency response center immediately.

HOW TO CALL

Find out what phone number to use for office hours and after hours. Some offices have a "triage" system where phone emergencies are called in and someone is appointed to call you back. Some offices have an automatic voice messaging/prompt system, which allows you to access someone by selecting a certain choice, even in emergencies.

DON'T WAIT

If you have been experiencing problems with your blood glucose for a couple of days, don't wait until Friday night to call the after-hours support person. You may end up being connected to someone who is not familiar with your history and not associated with your regular crew. Don't get mad if they require additional information (asking question upon question) from you in these situations. They are trying to do their best to make the right assessment of the situation, and they need your cooperation to get the right information.

THE EMERGENCY ROOM IS NOT A SUBSTITUTE FOR YOUR REGULAR OFFICE VISITS

It is important to stay on course with regular visits to prevent problems. If you run out of medication because of your lack of planning or knowledge of self-care, the emergency care center may cost you a fair amount of money, and you may still be referred back to your usual health care professional when they open the next day. Therefore, plan ahead for prescription renewals, attend classes to learn how to deal with problems, and keep regular appointments to avoid a Saturday-night trip to the local emergency room.

BE PREPARED TO ANSWER QUESTIONS

If you do need to call your doctor, be ready to answer the following common questions:

■ What type of diabetes do you have?

- What is your current blood glucose?
- When was the last reading (blood glucose) taken, and what was it?
- What medications did you take today?
- What medications are you taking for your diabetes management (actual name, dose, and timing)?
- What have you eaten today? Can you hold down food?
- Do you currently have a fever? For how long?
- What is your pharmacy's name and phone number?
- What is your insurance company and policy number? (If you have secondary insurance, you will need the information on both.)
- What are your symptoms and complaints?
- Do you feel you need an appointment, or just need to ask a question?
- What available phone number can you be reached at? (You may want to give a backup number of a family member or a friend if the information is urgent. Keep the phone on and available to receive the return call.)
- If you feel you need to go in for a sudden visit, have you arranged transportation so that the appointment time can be made accordingly?

MORE RESOURCES TO EXPLORE

BOOKS

Diabetes A to Z: What You Need to Know About Diabetes—Simply Put, 5th edition. American Diabetes Association; Alexandria, VA. 2003.

YOU—The Smart Patient: An Insider's Handbook for Getting the Best Treatment, by Michael F. Rozen and Mehmet C. Oz, with The Joint Commission. Free Press; New York, NY. 2006.

How to work with your insurance company

Even though most people have had some complaint about their health insurance company at some point, they should consider themselves lucky. Millions of individuals do not have the luxury of having medical insurance in the U.S., even today. If you have diabetes, you will be utilizing your insurance benefits throughout your lifetime. You will need coverage for simple needs such as blood glucose meter strips, diagnostic exams, and, possibly, hospitalizations. Policies and plans vary from person to person, but all insurance companies share certain common characteristics. The best way to have a positive experience with your insurance company is to be well informed. This section is filled with tips that should help.

■ **Do your research.** Before choosing a a health insurance plan, research your options well. Make decisions based not just on your health as of today, but what you anticipate your needs may be in the future. There may not be a perfect plan, but look at your needs, and the costs and access to services associated with each plan.

- **Curl up with a good policy.** Familiarize yourself with your policy. Even though the brochures and paperwork they give you when you enroll are overwhelming, pour yourself a cup of tea, stretch out, and read every word. It is important to know the rules and guidelines to avoid frustrations later.
- **Stay in the loop.** Read the policy updates you receive at work in the mail and stay current—most policies undergo several changes during the year. It is tempting to toss these updates, or file them in a drawer, but make the effort to read them. Some insurance companies offer special services such as pregnancy information kits, health fair screenings, informational lectures, health information pamphlets, and more. Since you are paying your dues, take advantage of every opportunity.
- **Know the little teeny-tiny phone number on the back of your card.** Call the customer service phone number for questions. This service is meant to answer your questions and help you navigate the health care system. Have your card with you when you call, and be prepared to spend some time on the phone. Very often, the customer service centers use automated voice messaging prompts to guide you to the right department. Make the call on a day when you have peace and quiet (no barking dogs in the background to raise your stress level) and when you have time (not when you have an upcoming appointment in 30 minutes across town). You may be on hold periodically as they route your call—use these minutes to file your bills, dust the living room, or water your plants.
- **Take it with you.** Keep your insurance cards with you, not at home. If you tend to lose things, make a copy (front and back) to keep at home in a safe place—just in case.
- **Let go of the past.** Don't keep old cards past their expiration dates—you can confuse which card is which. Cut up old cards to protect your privacy before tossing them in the trash. Provide current cards to all health care providers and pharmacies, ideally before your next visit or claim.

■ **Create a file**. Keep statements and receipts in a known area. You may need them to work through authorization processes, claims processes, or, yes, even appeals.

■ **Don't take short cuts.** If you wish to appeal a claim, follow the insurance company's directions completely and within the timeline they require. Trying to skip steps or bypass procedures will decrease your chances of having a successful appeal.

■ **Save the pretty stationery.** Use the proper forms when requested to get your paperwork processed quickly and correctly the first time.

■ **Be a pack-rat**. Keep copies of EVERYTHING you submit in the mail. Having this backup gives you the opportunity to be prepared in case the insurance company wishes to go over documents with you in the future. If you use a fax machine, choose a fax machine that prints out a confirmation of receipt message.

■ **Take names**. Write down first and last names and titles (job titles, not royal titles) of representatives when you talk to them each time. Some organizations are large, so just knowing "Sue helped me" may not be useful if you are trying to resolve a problem with a separate division. Keep a notepad by the phone, and politely ask them for their identity and title each time you talk. Add the time and date of the call to confirm your records. If you are having problems and need an advocate, contact your State Insurance Commissioner's Office for advice.

■ **Prepare for open enrollment days**. During open enrollment at your workplace, ask insurance company representatives to explain options and provide you with a directory of providers in advance, so you know your choices in terms of physicians, pharmacies, hospitals, diagnostic centers, etc.

■ **Beware of "outsiders."** If you are going to use a provider who is "outside" of your preferred providers, find out in advance how you'll need to process your claim if your plan will provide partial payment. In addition, some insurance companies partner with specific blood glucose meter companies for better pricing—if you use the preferred meter, you may save some money. Be cautious about taking free meters at health fairs, though, as your insurance company may limit your choices in terms of coverage for strips. Many times out-of-network providers/products will mean out-of-pocket payment from you, up to 100% of the charges. Terms for these providers/products are provided in the policy statement—the little booklet you were supposed to read.

▌ **Pre-authorization means pre-pare.** Ask your health care providers to perform and complete pre-authorization or notification requirements in advance of appointments and procedures.

▌ **Making transitions.** Update doctor's offices, pharmacies, and other health care providers when you have a name change, phone number change, address change, or policy change. In these days of cell phones and work transitions, many people change numbers frequently. If you make a change, notify everyone.

▌ **Start Monday mornings.** Plan ahead—make inquiry calls as soon as you can. Ideally, call the first of the week, as it may take a day or two to get the information back to you.

▌ **Check with new doctors.** If you are thinking of changing physicians or pharmacies, check with them to see if they accept your insurance before you make the move.

▌ **Know your generic drugs.** Remember which drugs are likely only covered as generic versions on your medication policy so that you are not surprised by substitutions. If you must have the trade-name version, find out what you need from your physician to justify the extra expense. If not approved, you will likely have to pay a higher co-pay for trade-name versions.

▌ **Renew early.** Renew prescriptions BEFORE you run out. This goes for medications, as well as testing supplies, pump supplies, and other health supplies. Many people obtain prescriptions through mail-order services, rather than the local drug store. These services may take several days to process renewals, so don't be caught without your meds.

▌ **Remember your manners.** Be patient when working with others; it may take time for things to be processed. To reduce your tension, ask representatives, "When should I expect to...," which gives them accountability and simultaneously creates a timeline to go on. Of course, don't let them forget about you—call back if the call is not returned by the timeline you both established.

MORE RESOURCES TO EXPLORE

MAGAZINES, JOURNALS, AND OTHER PUBLICATIONS

Choosing and Using a Health Plan. Agency for Health Care Policy and Research. U.S. Dept of Health and Human Services; AHCPR Publication No. 97-0011.

BOOKS

The Johns Hopkins Guide to Diabetes—For Today and Tomorrow, by CD Saudek, RR Rubin, and CS Shump. The Johns Hopkins University Press; Baltimore, MD. 1997.

WEBSITES

Agency for Healthcare Research
    and Quality . . . . WWW.AHRQ.GOV/CONSUMER/INSURANCEQA

CHAPTER 2
MAKE FINGER STICKS WORTH IT

How to make sticking your finger worth it

One day, a method may be created so that people with diabetes no longer have to prick or pierce their body parts to obtain blood glucose readings. Until that time, you'll need to make use of the devices that are on the market now.

It may be hard to appreciate the blood glucose meters of today, but they have come a long way. In the 1980s, most people were testing their urine to determine blood glu-cose levels, because meters were still in their infancy and not covered by insurance. Individuals would collect urine in a container, add special chemi-cals, shake or stir, and have to carefully time the testing procedure, only to get a "color" result that had to be compared to a color chart for interpretation. The ranges were varied, and the testing was, at best, awkward and not always accurate. So, despite your reserva-tions about testing, know that things have come a long way and that with a glucose meter, you currently have the fastest and most accurate way to control your diabetes.

A FINGER STICK COST/BENEFIT ANALYSIS

Testing your blood glucose is not generally a pleasant experience. But consider the following points when trying to determine whether finger-stick testing is worth it.

YOU CAN BE PROVEN RIGHT

Who doesn't like to be right? It can certainly boost your ego. If you have had diabetes for a while, you may feel like you can predict your blood glucose (within 5 mg/dl, of course) without even removing your meter from its case. This is a special gift, but it's a gift you need to verify, especially since symptoms of high or low blood glucose can become less noticeable with time. Prove yourself right and test to confirm.

IT IS A GOOD EXCUSE FOR A 5-MINUTE BREAK

Most meters provide a test result in as few as 5 seconds. However, no one at work needs to know that. Tell your coworkers it takes 5 minutes and make it seem like an inconvenience. A small break seems like a just reward for a deed well done.

IT IS A CONVERSATION STARTER

> A nice dinner can be ruined by fretting, as each bite makes you think, "I wonder what *this* will do to my blood glucose?"

If you pull out a blood glucose meter in front of friends, it is sure to get the questions going. Be honest about what you are doing. Diabetes is a growing epidemic; you might learn that someone else has diabetes and can be a future source of support or camaraderie. Talk about how diabetes affects you, so everyone can understand diabetes better.

ENJOY A MEAL IN PEACE

A nice dinner can be ruined by fretting, as each bite makes you think, "I wonder what *this* will do to my blood glucose?" Stop fretting and test to find out. Ideally, test before a meal and 2 hours after to see what effect the food and/ or your medication has on your blood glucose.

Depending on some other factors, you can expect about a 40–60 mg/dl difference from a pre-meal blood glucose reading and a reading 2 hours after a meal. If the difference is larger than this, it could mean:

▌ Overall, you ate more than you expected
▌ Your food may have contained hidden fat, carbohydrate, or calories
▌ You ate a meal with a moderate to high fat level, causing a delayed rise in your blood glucose
▌ Your diabetes medications may need to be adjusted
▌ Your nutrition plans needs review
▌ You need more information from a registered dietitian on foods

GET A GOOD NIGHT'S REST

High blood glucose levels usually mean more trips to the bathroom. Not only is this inconvenient for you, but it disturbs other members of the household as well. If you test often, you maybe able to identify high blood glucose levels at certain times. Take this information to your health care team so that your management plan (and/or medications) can be adjusted. Good control means less hyperglycemia, and fewer symptoms like getting up in the middle of the night. Lack of sleep can make you feel tired, stressed, and even depressed. Everyone needs their ZZZs.

PROTECT YOURSELF AND YOUR FAMILY

Unstable blood glucose levels can cause unclear thinking or poor choices. Having high or low blood glucose behind the wheel of a car can lead to disastrous results—especially if your family is with you. You should definitely check your blood glucose when:

▌ Driving long distances
▌ Being alone with children in your care
▌ Traveling alone or with others
▌ Working with dangerous equipment
▌ Being "off" your usual daily schedule

ENSURE YOU TAKE THE RIGHT AMOUNT OF MEDICATION

There are quite a few diabetes medications, insulin especially, that need to be timed to meals *and* based on your blood glucose readings. Medications are expensive and have been prescribed to improve your control. Don't waste your money—test your blood glucose to know the right amount of medication to take.

LESS HYPOGLYCEMIA

Checking your glucose often can teach you how your body reacts to different activities and situations. If you take insulin or an oral medication that can cause hypoglycemia, this knowledge can help you prepare and prevent severe low blood glucose levels. No one likes hypoglycemia. Testing can help you also identify when your blood glucose may be sliding down and allow you to take measures to prevent hypoglycemia immediately.

BE A SUCCESS STORY

You can brag all you want about how well you control your diabetes, but you need the numbers to prove it. How often you test is up to you and your health care team, but be sure you that once you have a plan of action, you stick to it. You may also need to adjust your schedule or check more often, especially if you are changing therapy, pregnant, nursing, using an insulin pump, or traveling. It is OK to miss a check once in a while, but stay determined to perform recommended testing. Your management choices will help define your future health.

MORE RESOURCES TO EXPLORE

WEBSITES

American Diabetes Association . . . . WWW.DIABETES.ORG

How to choose a blood glucose meter

Not everyone with diabetes needs to check his or her blood glucose multiple times throughout the day. In fact, depending on the advice of your health care team, you may not need to check all that often. Then again, if you're on an insulin pump, you may need to check your glucose several times a day. No matter what your regimen, though, it still makes sense for almost everyone with diabetes to have a blood glucose meter. Even if you check only occasionally, knowing your blood glucose level gives you vital information to make appropriate decisions and take actions, if necessary.

There are many types of blood glucose meters available on the market. Just like everything else, there are a variety of options and features. Choosing the right one for you can take a little preparation and homework.

THINGS TO CONSIDER

With all of the choices available, there are a few things you should keep in mind once you begin shopping for a meter.

AISLE
5
Blood Sugar
Meters

FIND OUT WHAT METER IS COVERED ON YOUR PLAN

Generally, home meter costs are at least partially covered by health insurance plans, if not in full. Some insurance plans have contracts with only certain meter companies and consider devices from these companies "preferred" choices. If your insurance policy has a contract such as this and you don't pick the "preferred" brand, you may be in for a higher co-payment—not just for the meter, but for the strips as well. If you expect you will pay some of the cost of the meter, ask your health care providers for rebate coupons or about discounts the company may be offering. Check out diabetes-related magazines for special offers in the advertising pages. Compare costs between hometown pharmacies as well; there can be a sizable difference.

DON'T FORGET ABOUT STRIPS

Remember you will also be purchasing strips on a regular basis, so if you are given a choice of products, compare costs of the strips, as well as what stores carries what strips. Most of the larger pharmacies stock a variety of test-strip brands, but some smaller pharmacies do not. Save yourself driving across town for strips; check into availability first.

WARRANTY

Pick a device that has a warranty, preferably for at least 3 years. This information should be printed on the box, or a pharmacist/health care provider should be able to find out for you. Meters have a life expectancy of about 3–5 years, but use and abuse over that period of time can shorten its lifespan. Frequent testers and travelers may want to consider a change every few years due to the wear and tear. A lifetime warranty is not usually a high priority, however, since meters continue to improve and chances are you will want to upgrade in the future.

CARRYING CASES

If you're going to be testing frequently, you're going to have your meter with you much of the time. Pick a size that will allow you to comfortably carry the meter and the necessary testing supplies (lancet, strips, etc.). Some of the cases will only hold the meter, and will require a second case or container for testing supplies.

FEATURES

All meters will give you a blood glucose result—but is that all you need or want? Some diabetes magazines and websites offer product guides each year and will compare products. Manufacturer websites will offer information about their product and, often, online demon-

A WORD ABOUT FREE GIVEAWAY METERS

When offered a free glucose meter, a person generally thinks three things: Free! Free! Free! While there is no denying that the price is right, there are other things to consider.

▌Check to make sure strips for this meter are covered by your insurance plan; if not, this "free" meter may actually cost you more in the long run.

▌Check to see if it is an older model—some of the newer meters have better features. Also consider that less expensive meters do not have the same durability or quality parts, and they may not last as long as more expensive devices.

▌While you may not have to pay money, free meters often still have a cost. Many times you'll be asked to provide personal information or sign up for a service or an additional purchase to receive your free meter. Be very careful what you commit to—read the fine print, and ask questions.

strations so you can check out a meter before buying. Keep in mind that, overall, most blood glucose meters generally have similar steps and provide quick results, but have some different features and looks. These features are discussed below.

BLOOD GLUCOSE METER FEATURE COMPARISONS—PROS AND CONS

There are many features offered by today's advanced technology meters. Following is a summary of some things to consider.

FEATURE: AUTOMATIC CALIBRATION

How does it benefit me?   Every batch of blood glucose test strips produced at the factory comes out a bit different. Before using a strip from a new package, most meters require you to perform step(s) so your meter can properly recognize the new batch of strips. This is called "calibration" or "coding," and it is often done using code numbers or letters, or code chips. If your meter requires calibration, you need to perform these steps with every new package of strips, which is an obvious inconvenience. A meter with automatic calibration takes care of this for you.

Any drawbacks? You probably won't be able to use generic strips, otherwise, there aren't many drawbacks. Automatic calibration is a good thing.

FEATURE: ALTERNATIVE-SITE TESTING ABILITY

How does it benefit me? Alternative-site testing means you can test (stick) yourself at areas other than your fingertips. If you often use the computer, do needlecraft work, play a musical instrument, or work in a health care profession, you may welcome the opportunity to give your fingertips a rest. Areas for alternative-site testing usually include the palm, forearm, and thigh.

Any drawbacks? Because of differences in skin thickness, blood flow, and sensitivity, alternative-site testing does not work for everyone. For low blood glucose levels or extremely high blood glucose levels, some health care professionals recommended using finger-stick testing to confirm readings, as there can be differences in the results due to how blood flows throughout the body.

FEATURE: MEMORY

How does it benefit me? The memory feature in most blood glucose monitors saves previous readings to an internal drive. If you write down your blood glucose in your glucose diary every single time, you are a rare individual. Having a memory is great as a backup for those times when you don't or can't write down a reading.

Any drawbacks? Even with a "memory" meter, you still need to write down your numbers. When the memory gets full, it will usually discard the oldest reading. Also, the date and time must be set up correctly for the information to be useful—so don't forget to adjust for daylight saving dates!

FEATURE: DATA MANAGEMENT FEATURES

How does it benefit me? Some meters will allow you to see your daily, seven-day, fourteen-day, or thirty-day blood glucose average with the touch of a button, which may help you visualize your overall control. In addition, some meters allow you to mark results with notations, such as pre-meal, post-meal, with medication, without medication, etc. Most meters with data management features can also upload data to computers.

Any drawbacks?   Just as with the memory feature, you can begin to rely on your data management feature too much. You still need to write down your readings. When the memory gets full, it will usually discard the oldest reading. Uploading your data will also sometimes erase the memory, so make sure you print out the results after uploading, be it at home or at your doctor's office. Data management features may also affect the battery life of your meter (though helping you identify trends, problems, and successes is well worth the cost of a AAA battery). Some of the advanced features look great, but are only useful if you are willing to take the extra time to input the information when testing.

FEATURE: SMALL SIZE, LIGHTWEIGHT

How does it benefit me?   Portability.

Any drawbacks?   Losing the little guy. Little meters may also have odd-sized batteries, as opposed to the more standard AA or AAA you will find in larger meters. And don't forget you still need to be able to read the screen and work the buttons.

FEATURE: BROAD TESTING RANGE (FOR EXAMPLE, 20–600 MG/DL)

How does it benefit me?   The range indicates how well the meter performs at different glucose levels. Most meters offer a broad enough range to capture your daily readings.

Any drawbacks?   A meter with a narrow testing range may produce an error message when it is unable to read a glucose result out of its range (though this may be a technique error, so always try again). Generally, the broader the range, the better.

FEATURE: BATTERIES

How does it benefit me?   It is easier to find standard AA and AAA batteries—especially on sale—than unique batteries. These standard batteries are also more likely to be available in a rechargeable format.

Any drawbacks?   Meters that use standard batteries are usually larger and bulkier. Conversely, small batteries are sometimes difficult to insert if you have arthritis or neuropathy. And again, odd-sized batteries may be hard to find, especially when you really need one on a Saturday night.

FEATURE: INCLUDED LANCET DEVICE

How does it benefit me?   Lancet devices, the object used to prick your finger for a drop of blood, generally come with a meter. Some lancet devices have adjustable depth guides, so you can pick a depth that is comfortable to you. Lancets may also have different end caps for alternative-site testing capabilities. Some devices have automatic triggers and needle removal features, which can help with loading and unloading.

Any drawbacks?   Some lancet devices use only name-brand lancets, while others use a more generic size. There is not one perfect lancet device for all persons—skin thickness, sensitivity, and blood flow issues influence the outcome of the use of the device. If you don't like the lancet that comes with your meter, you might have to purchase a lancet sold by another company to find one that gives you the results you need and the comfort you deserve.

MORE RESOURCES TO EXPLORE

MAGAZINES, JOURNALS, AND PERIODICALS

Diabetes Forecast—Resource Guide 2009
Every year, *Diabetes Forecast*, the magazine of the American Diabetes Association, produces a Resource Guide with the latest information on meters, lancets, insulins, medications, and much more.

WEBSITES

Abbott Laboratories	WWW.ABBOTTDIABETESCARE.COM
Bayer Health Care	WWW.BAYERDIABETES.COM
Home Diagnostics	WWW.HOMEDIAGNOSTICS.COM
Johnson and Johnson	WWW.LIFESCAN.COM
Roche Diagnostics	WWW.ACCU-CHECK.COM
Sanvita Inc.	WWW.SANVITA.COM

How to use your blood glucose meter

Whether you use a simple blood glucose meter or a model with lots of bells and whistles, you will become an expert in how to use it in a very short time. Before using it the first time, however, it is best to have someone walk you through the process in person. Give yourself plenty of time for this first test, and pick an environment with good light and a work surface. Try to stay relaxed. And if all else fails, read the user's manual.

GENERAL METER TIPS

HANDLE WITH CARE

A good rule of thumb: treat your meter as you would your mobile phone. It should not get wet, be handled roughly, or be left exposed to extreme temperatures. Most blood glucose meters have a functional temperature range for performance; in other words, they should be used and stored at certain temperatures. Usually this is room temperature. So it would not be wise to leave your meter in a closed car during a hot summer day in Georgia. After this baking, it may still turn on, but there may be damage to the screen or other parts that could affect its use.

> " If all else fails, read the user's manual. "

CLEANING

Blood glucose meters should be kept clean by using a soft cloth to remove dirt or debris. Avoid using harsh cleaning agents. A washcloth moistened with water should easily remove dirt on the device and screen. Alcohol and other liquid cleaning agents may streak the display window, or could seep into seams of the device and cause internal damage.

MORE POWER, SCOTTY!

Keep working batteries in your meter at all times. Some meters will have a battery life indicator or flash a warning message when the battery is getting low. It would be a good idea to keep an extra new battery on hand, or in the meter travel case. Rechargeable batteries may be an option, but some manufacturers suggest they not be used—check your user's manual to be sure. Once again, keep your hand-written glucose log up to date! If your meter loses power, it will probably also lose all of the data being stored in the memory.

WARRANTY

With your new meter, take the time to fill out the warranty post-card included in your meter kit, and then send it in. This will register your device with the company so you will be notified of any recalls, problems, or special offers.

CHECKING YOUR BLOOD GLUCOSE WITH YOUR METER: THE BASIC STEPS

1. ASSEMBLE YOUR SUPPLIES.

Before you start, wash your hands with soap and water. Dry your hands with a paper towel or clean towel, rather than the used towel that has been hanging in the bathroom all week. Be sanitary. Make sure you have all of the materials you'll need, including:

- Meter laid on a flat surface
- Test strips (that have not expired)
- Cotton ball
- Lancet device loaded with a new lancet (while some people reuse lancets, it can be less comfortable and less sterile than using a new one each time)

TIPS ON CLEANING

Antibacterial soap and water is the preferred method for cleaning a test site. Dry the area with a paper towel or let it air dry—no wiping or blowing germs and dust onto the area. Alcohol pads are fine to use, but if you have dry skin or irritated cuticles the alcohol may cause further drying and possible cracking. Additionally, the alcohol must be completely dry, or else you might end up knowing the glucose level of a mixture of alcohol and blood.

Antibacterial hand sanitizers should not be used to clean sites for blood glucose testing. These products may contain other chemicals, perfumes, or additives that could possibly give a false reading. Stick with plain ol' soap and water.

2. TURN ON THE METER AND FOLLOW INSTRUCTIONS.

Follow the manufacturer's directions for turning on your meter. If you plan to use the memory, ensure that the time and date are set correctly. Make sure you are not seeing any errors or problems on the screen. If the screen display is faint or blinking, consult the user's manual to identify the problem—you may need a new battery, or it may be a sign of electrical malfunction. If you get an error message, once again, consult the user's manual before testing or call the toll-free customer support number written on the back of the device for help. If the meter is having a problem, chances are the test result will not be accurate, so wait until the problem is resolved. You may also have to calibrate (set your meter to interpret the test strip results). Read your instruction booklet or call the manufacturer's toll-free help number to learn how to do this important step.

3. INSERT A NEW TEST STRIP.

Follow the manufacturer's instructions for inserting a strip. Handle the test strips with care, making sure they do not get wet or handled in the testing area before being inserted into the device. Do not use a strip that has fallen in the sink or been left out for more than few minutes.

4. PREPARE AND PRICK.

Prepare the testing site by increasing circulation for better blood flow. If you are testing your fingers, shake your fingers or pump your hand into a fist a few times. If you are using alternative-site testing, you may be instructed to rub the area to increase blood flow. Cold tissue may not have good blood flow—warm up the area before testing if you have been exposed to cold temperatures.

Prick the site with the lancet device. Once again, follow the manufacturer's directions for using the lancet. To make testing more comfortable, try different sites to see what works best for you.

If you do not get the quantity you need, "milk" the finger by using your other hand to squeeze from the base of your finger to the tip. Hold your fingertip down (not up in the air) to let gravity help. Relax the finger—constricting the finger or being tense will restrict blood flow to the area. If you use your fingertips often (e.g., needle crafters, computer keyboarders, ball players, brick layers, musicians) and have tough skin, you may want to use the fourth or fifth fingers, which may be more supple.

FOR ALTERNATIVE-SITE TESTING

If you're using a meter that allows alternative-site testing, follow the manufacturer's directions and remember that getting a sample may take a little more time. The most important tip is timing—do not release pressure on the lancet device until the appropriate time has expired. Be patient; allow sufficient time for the sample to appear.

---

5. APPLY THE SAMPLE TO THE RECEIVING PART OF THE STRIP.

Too much blood may cause a false reading or error message to occur. Too little blood may cause a false reading, with the result being lower than your actual blood glucose count. Some strips can be reapplied if the first contact did not sufficiently coat the receiving part of the strip. Before trying a reapplication, read your user's manual to find out if this is acceptable.

Blot the site with a cotton ball with slight pressure until bleeding stops. If you are a heavy bleeder or on blood-thinning medications, you may want to have several cotton balls on hand. You may also want to use a low-depth setting with your lancet device. If you bruise easy, try to wiggle your finger soon after the stick to encourage blood circulation. A bandage is usually not necessary unless you'd simply like to avoid getting blood on your clothes or other surfaces.

6. RECORD YOUR RESULT IN A BLOOD GLUCOSE DIARY.

If you did not get a diary from your meter company or your health care professional, make your own with a small spiral notebook. Record the time, date, and result. Make notes for any usual events such as illness, pain, skipped meals, special meals, missed medications, etc.

7. WRAPPING IT UP:

▌Remove and discard the used test strip.
▌Remove the used lancet and discard in a sharps container or approved disposal container.
  ▌A sharps container is designed specifically to hold needles and syringes and can be purchased from a pharmacy, though mail order, or online. Check with the waste-removal system or company that serves your neighborhood about safe disposal of sharps. They may want you to contain the sharps or identify them so that waste-removal company workers do not get injured. See Thing to Know 43 for more on sharps disposal.
▌Store the meter and test strips as recommended.
  ▌For storage, manufacturers usually recommend a room temperature area (not a steamy bathroom or hot kitchen), out of direct sunlight, and away from the blast of forced air (heat system or air-conditioning).
▌Check your supplies.
▌If you are running low, get a refill on your prescription or supplies in the next day or two. Don't put it off; you might need more than you anticipate for unexpected blood glucose swings or events.
▌Pat yourself on the back.
▌Your health care team may ask you to check your glucose, but, unfortunately, they will not be able to thank you or

congratulate you each time you test. Develop your own personal reward system for keeping up with regular testing. A professional car wash once a month or a night out at the movies can be nice treats.

HAVING PROBLEMS?

If you have any problems with your meter, consult the customer service number on the back of the meter, especially if you are getting repeated error messages. Customer service may be able to talk you through the problem. If you need visual assistance on how to do the test, ask for a video or DVD of the instructions to be sent to you. A certified diabetes educator can also meet with you individually to help you with the process. Sometimes it is easier to have someone guide you through it the first time to give you tips along the way and boost your confidence.

Remember, if you're having a problem, there is help available. You simply need to ask. Asking for help is a better solution than stuffing away your meter in a drawer out of frustration. It can't do you any good there.

9

How to get a good drop of blood the first time

It can seem very intimidating to stick you own finger for blood glucose testing. For some, the fear of sticking a finger vanishes after a few blood glucose checks, while for others, hesitation persists for some time. Until manufacturers come up with a needle-less lancet device that is affordable and useful, a glucose check will involve a needle prick. Fortunately, there are special techniques you can use to help with comfort. Plus, if your technique is good, you can get a good drop of blood the first time, which means fewer finger sticks.

If you want to improve your glucose check technique, focus on four general practices: picking the right site, preparing the site, performing the stick, and maintaining sites for ongoing use.

PICKING THE RIGHT SITE

FOR FINGER-STICK TESTING

Finger-stick testing is generally performed on the four fingers, but not the thumb. Hold one of your fingers in front of you and imagine a horseshoe drawn around the tip, with the horseshoe pointing down. These are the recommended areas for finger-stick testing.

Tips:

- ▌ Don't prick beyond the first knuckle (or finger crease).
- ▌ Either side of the finger is fine to use.
- ▌ Stay away from your fingernail bed.

- Alternate fingers and sites so that the sites do not become sore or covered with scar tissue.
- If you use your fingertips often and have toughened skin (e.g., needle crafters, computer keyboarders, athletes, musicians, construction workers), you may want to use the fourth or fifth fingers, which may have more supple skin.

FOR ALTERNATIVE-SITE TESTING

Consult your user's manual for approved areas. The following areas are often approved areas for testing:

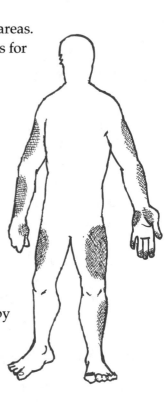

- Upper front of forearm
- Thigh and calf
- Outside edge of hand
- Inside ball of thumb

Tips:

- Avoid areas with heavy body hair, since the sample might get caught in the hair.
- Avoid areas with calloused or cracked skin.
- Avoid areas around scars and tattoos by at least 1–2 inches.
- Avoid areas near wounds or rashes.
- Change sites often so you don't bruise or develop scar tissue.
- If you think you are currently experiencing a low blood glucose reaction or if in the past your symptoms have not matched results from alternative-site testing, use the finger-stick method instead.

PREPARING THE SITE

This was discussed briefly in the previous section, but preparing the site can lead to better results. There are two things to do:

- Clean the site with soap and water and allow to completely dry

▌ Get blood moving to the site:
  ▌ **Fingers**—make a fist several times, shake out your hand a few times, lower your hand below your waist, or rinse your hands in warm water.
  ▌ **Alternative sites**—rub or massage the area with your hand for a few seconds.

PERFORMING THE STICK

USE THE LANCET DEVICE CORRECTLY

▌ Read the manual or watch a demonstration to see how your lancet device is used. Not positioning the lancet firmly on the target area is the most common culprit for not getting a good stick on the first try. A light touch may not allow the lancet to penetrate the skin as deeply as it is intended to.

▌ The "snap" of the trigger is an audible noise in most devices and can cause a sudden reflex reaction to pull away. Not only can this cause a poor stick, it can also tear more tissue than intended, leading to more, not less, pain. Lancets are made to self-retract immediately after the trigger is engaged within the lancing device. So don't worry: it won't stick you twice.

▌ Make sure the depth is set correctly on your lancet device. Try the middle-depth setting first. If you get too little blood, turn the setting the next time to a deeper depth. If you get too much, turn the setting down to the next choice.

▌ Some lancet devices offer alternative-site testing capabilities. Follow the manufacturer's directions carefully for these devices. You may need to use a special protective cap on the device for this type of testing.

▌ Use a quality lancet for the device. Some less expensive lancets may not provide the same level of comfort or success. Using lancets more than once can be more painful and less sterile.

THE STICK

For finger testing:

▌ Use *gentle* pressure and squeeze your finger to obtain enough blood.

- If you do not immediately get the amount you need, use your other hand to "milk" the blood down by performing a continuous squeezing motion that starts at the base of your finger and ends at the fingertip.
- Hold the finger down (not up in the air) to let gravity help.
- Relax your finger. Constricting or tensing your finger will likely restrict blood flow to the area. Take a deep breath.
- Work quickly so that the meter does not "time out."
- Apply the blood per the meter manufacturer's guidelines.

For alternative-site testing:

- If you are using a lancet device with an adjustable depth, turn the setting up to the *highest* setting the first time, and see if it produces a sufficient sample.
- Hold the lancet device on the site long enough to allow enough time for the blood to seep out (check your user's manual for the recommended time). Blood comes out easier and quicker for a finger-stick test than with alternative-site testing. This is normal, so be willing to wait.
- Experiment with different sites for comfort and blood flow.
- Work quickly so that the meter does not "time out."
- Apply the blood per the meter manufacturer's guidelines.
- If the process does not work for you (and for some it won't due to skin thickness, circulation, and other individual issues), you don't have to return the meter. Simply follow the directions for finger-stick testing instead.
- Talk to an educator about alternative-site testing; they may have tips that make the procedure successful for you.

MAINTAINING SITES FOR ONGOING USE

You want to be sure that you do not overuse a site. In addition to rotating sites, there are additional steps you can take to ensure check your blood glucose remains comfortable and successful for years to come.

- Exercise—keep the blood moving!
- Don't smoke—smoking will impair your circulation.
- Use lotion regularly, to keep your skin supple.
- When doing household tasks such as dishwashing, cleaning,

and other chores, wear kitchen gloves to keep water or chemicals from drying out your fingers.

▎Wear garden or work gloves when working with tools or equipment.

▎Avoid tight-fitting jewelry on your fingers.

▎Be sure to take any prescribed medications for heart or circulation problems.

MORE RESOURCES TO EXPLORE

WEBSITES

Food and Drug Administration. . . . . WWW.FDA.GOV/CDRH/CDRHHHC
The Food and Drug Administration, through the CDRH Home Health Care Committee division, offers a guide, Blood Glucose Meters—Getting the Most Out of Your Meter, *that can be downloaded in PDF form from this website.*

How to write a useful logbook

If you are going to take the time to test, make sure your efforts aren't in vain: write down the result each time. You can keep these records in a logbook (or log, or blood glucose diary, or diabetes diary). What form this logbook takes is up to you. You more than likely received a little book of rows and columns with your meter kit, but a spiral notebook, or even letter-sized pages you print from your computer will work as well.

This section will show you how to make your little logbook useful in managing your diabetes. You may have been told to write the results down, but not necessarily told how you can use it to solve problems.

THE ESSENTIAL ELEMENTS OF A LOGBOOK

August 21st

Dear Diary,
When I got out of the bed, I discovered the dog had taken off with my slipper. After a brief chase around the house, I recovered the wet slipper (dog slobber) and put it on my foot. I decided to let the dog outside, and when I did, he saw the neighbor's cat and took off after it with paws flying—right through my flower garden. The cat was not particularly bright, and chose to jump on the roof of my new convertible car. The dog, straight from his dash through the begonias, followed and leaped repeatedly on the car with his muddy paws and claws. The cat reacted by digging her claws into the canvas top of my convertible and hissing back while I...

When you think of a log or diary, you may think of the above. Thankfully, you do not have to write a huge chapter every time you test. Instead, stick to the essential elements:

❚ Date
❚ Time
❚ Relation to a meal (before or after)
❚ Blood glucose reading
❚ Notes (for detailing special circumstances)

So, instead of the paragraph listed above, it could be noted like this:

Date	Time	Before or After Meal	Blood Glucose (mg/dl)	Notes
6/4/07	7:43 am	Before	56	Exercise and stress before breakfast. Treated low with 4 oz juice, retested at 8 a.m., now 97, ate breakfast

THE TINY, IMPORTANT "NOTES" SECTION

The "Notes" column is often very tiny in preprinted logbooks, but these details are important, so fit in as much as you can. This information can help you better analyze the circumstances contributing to your blood glucose, as well as the blood glucose levels that follow. If the Notes section is too small, find another logbook with more space, or create your own. When filling out the Notes section, some helpful details to note may include:

❚ Skipped meals
❚ Extra snack eaten
❚ New food eaten
❚ Amount of carbohydrate eaten
❚ Amount of medication taken
❚ Exercise (type and how long)
❚ PMS symptoms
❚ Menstrual cycle
❚ Special social events, such as parties or dinner out

- Everyday activities, such as walking the dog or gardening
- Illness
- Stress
- Off-routine events (late meal, slept late)
- Work schedule changes (day shift, night shift)
- New medication started

Some of these details may seem meaningless, but any of this can be used as evidence to solve the mystery of the unexpected blood glucose level. Without these notes, you may fall into the trap of feeling powerless about your blood glucose control. Don't let this happen! Information can help identify causes for swings or unusual events, and over the long run, it can help you determine trends.

STYLES OF LOGBOOKS

There are many styles of logbooks now available, some of which aren't technically books. A summary of some of the types available:

- Paper and pencil; you create on your own
- Preprinted logbooks from meter companies (who may send you new copies upon request) or publishers
- Preprinted diabetes diaries/calendars from diabetes supply companies
- Printed log sheets from health care professionals
- PC software from meter companies (usually only works with the brand of meter from that company) or private software companies (which will usually need to have the necessary hardware and software required for each meter brand)
- PDA software (allows you to enter data into your favorite PDA or even smart phones)
- Online programs (data is entered over the Internet)

TREND SPOTTING

Writing down your blood glucose readings is not just a homework assignment for the benefit of your health care professionals; *you* need to use this information as well. Review this information on your own to see if you see recurring changes or trends. You may notice things like:

- Your lowest reading is almost always at 4 PM in the afternoon.
- Your highest readings happen in the morning when you wake up.
- Your blood glucose levels after lunch are higher at work than on the weekends or off days.

Of course, these are just examples and every case will be difference. Identifying trends is not always easy and you may find it's more an art than a science. To help, try the following tips:

- Write down the results in the same format each time.
- Ideally, write the results in a column and row format so you can easily compare the same time between different days (see the example earlier in this section).
- Vary the times you test to provide the most information possible.
- Be honest; if you ate two donuts on a whim, write it down.

Once you have taken the information and possibly spotted some trends, take your facts and theories to your health care providers. Together, you may be able to come up with new strategies to resolve your problem areas.

TIMING—HOW OFTEN SHOULD YOU RECORD?

Ask your health care professional when and how often you should be testing. If you want to make the most of your logbook, try testing at various times each day. If you have been told to check twice a day, choose two of the following times each day and rotate between days:

- Fasting (before breakfast)
- 2 hours after breakfast
- Before lunch
- 2 hours after lunch
- Before supper
- 2 hours after supper
- Bedtime
- Midnight
- 3 A.M.

USING YOUR LOGBOOK— REAL WORLD EXAMPLES

You may already have questions about a certain event or challenging numbers you are experiencing regularly. Following are a few examples of situations you may face and how you might use blood glucose checks and your logbook to get to the bottom of some perplexing glucose readings.

HOW DOES EXERCISE AFFECT BLOOD GLUCOSE?

Follow these steps:

1. Test before the activity.
2. If your blood glucose is in your target range, continue. If not, wait until your blood glucose is more stable.
3. Test during the activity if it is longer than 1 hour.
4. Test after the activity.
5. Test hourly for at least 3 hours after the activity.

Before drawing any conclusions, perform these steps twice on nonconsecutive days for each type of exercise, as there are certainly day-to-day variances that may occur. However, it can help show you if you need a snack, and when, or if you don't.

DOES A HONEYBUN AFFECT BLOOD GLUCOSE?

Follow these steps:

1. Test before eating the item. If your blood glucose is in your target range, continue. If not, try when your blood glucose is more stable.
2. Eat only the item you are interested in.
3. Test 2 hours after eating.
4. Test 3 hours after eating.
5. Test 4 hours after eating.

Check your readings to see how much the food raises your glucose level and when the rise happens. If this is a food you want to include in your meal plan, take the information back to your health care professionals (ideally a RD or CDE) to see how you could work the food into your plan (portions, frequency, medication adjustments, etc.).

DOES PMS AFFECT MY BLOOD GLUCOSE?

Follow these steps:

1. Test four times a day at least three to four days before your cycle begins.
2. Test four times a day during your cycle.
3. Test four times a day one to two days after your cycle ends.
4. Repeat this process for at least two menstrual cycles and compare numbers.

Did you see changes during this time? Take the information back to your health care professionals. It is not uncommon to have medication adjustments or strategies for special days.

MORE RESOURCES TO EXPLORE

PRODUCTS

Diabetes Day-By-Day Planner
  This day-by-day planner can be ordered from
  WWW.MEDICALPUBLISHING.COM.

American Diabetes Association Blood Glucose Log Book
  This pocket-sized logbook contains entries for three months of readings. Includes extra room for notes, information on goals and pattern management, a food diary, and more.
  Can be ordered from HTTP://STORE.DIABETES.ORG.

Diabetes Pilot
  This diabetes management software, available for PCs and PDAs, tracks glucose readings, food intake, exercise, and much more. Available from WWW.DIABETESPILOT.COM.

Sugar Stats
  A browser-based diabetes management program. Offers a variety of tracking options and can be accessed anywhere with a web connection, though an account with the service is required.
  Available at WWW.SUGARSTATS.COM.

(continued)

(continued)

WEBSITES

American Diabetes Association . . . . WWW.DIABETES.ORG
  *The website of the American Diabetes Association contains much on blood
  glucose checks and pattern management, especially in the
  Youth Zone.*

Mendosa.com: Living with Diabetes . . . . WWW.MENDOSA.COM
  *This website by writer David Mendosa, who specializes in diabetes, contains
  one of the oldest and most comprehensive lists of diabetes resources on
  the Internet, including a section devoted entirely to software and diabetes
  management tools.*

CHAPTER 3
MAKE EVERY DAY GO BETTER

How to start the day

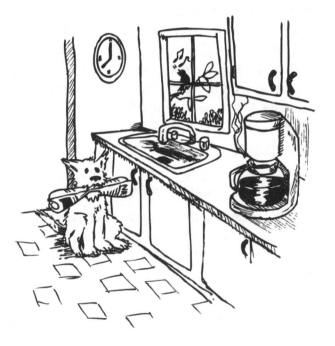

Most of us have some sort of morning routine. Some are rushed and some are relaxed. But often, our morning rituals set the tone for the rest of the day. Following is a prescription for a relaxing, productive, and healthy start every morning.

▮ When you wake up, take a minute to start the day with a positive thought. You may want to think about the opportunities ahead or simply daydream. Or you may want to write in a daily journal, or read a daily meditation, passage of poetry, or chapter of a book. In some way, start the day with a positive outlook.

▌ After rising, do a quick check of your house shoes or slippers before slipping your toes inside. Diabetes can cause nerve damage, and nerve damage can decrease sensation in your feet. Without normal feeling, you can unknowingly step on or into hazardous items in your footwear and walk around on it, which could cause a blister, cut, or pressure sore. Run your hand inside and inspect your slippers or shoes with your eyes before stepping in. Avoid going barefoot, even in the house. *Always* protect your feet against injury.

▌ If you're like most people, the bathroom is your first stop in the morning. Turn on the light to avoid tripping over a dropped towel or clothes on the floor. If your circulation is impaired or your blood glucose control is not on track, it can be more difficult to heal from a fall. Therefore, have a clear path to the bathroom, nightlights, and non-slip rugs on your floors.

▌ If your health care team asks that you check in the morning, assemble your supplies and test your blood glucose before breakfast for a "fasting" reading.

▌ Take a nice warm shower or bath, but avoid using very hot water. Uncontrolled glucose levels can lead to dry skin, due to the dehydrating effects of prolonged high blood glucose levels. See Thing to Know 22 for more information about bathing and showering.

▌ Apply a moisturizer after bathing, checking the condition of your skin while doing so. Choose a quality moisturizer for the best results.

▌ Check your feet after your bath or shower. Look for any changes in skin color, nail color, or skin condition. Check for any sensation changes. Use a cotton swab to touch the top, sides, bottom of your feet and note if you have any increased or decreased sensitivity. Report any problems with your feet to your health care professionals at once. See Thing to Know 36 for more information about foot care.

A HIGH READING IN THE MORNING— WHAT DOES IT MEAN?

For some individuals, morning fasting blood glucose levels may actually be higher than later in the day, which may make it a challenge to control blood glucose levels during eating hours. If you have high blood glucose levels in the morning, you may be experiencing one or more issues:

IF YOU HAVE TYPE 1 DIABETES

▌ A high number first thing in the morning may be the "dawn phenomenon," a change in hormone levels while you sleep that can cause blood glucose levels to rise on their own. This situation needs to be brought to your doctor's attention. Testing at bedtime, 2–3:00 A.M., and when rising for a few days in a row can help determine if you have dawn phenomenon.

▌ Sometimes you may unknowingly experience a low blood glucose during the night. Your body responds to this stress by releasing glucose from your stored energy supply back into your bloodstream. This is called the Somogyi effect. Checking your blood glucose before bed, at 2–3:00 A.M., and at 6:00 A.M. for a few days might help reveal a problem with nighttime hypoglycemia. Talk to your health care professional if you think you may have had this occur more than once.

IF YOU HAVE TYPE 2 DIABETES

▌ A high fasting number may indicate some insulin resistance, which is a common problem in type 2 diabetes. Fortunately, there are medications available to treat this condition. If your bedtime blood glucose is lower than your morning reading, it is important to discuss this with your doctor.

IF YOU ARE PREGNANT

▌ Hormones in pregnancy may also affect blood glucose levels in the morning and your target range may need to be adjusted to reflect this.

FOR ANY TYPE OF DIABETES

▌ Late-night meals, high-fat dinners, middle-of-the-night snacking, and digestive problems such as gastroparesis (slowed emptying of the stomach, a common complication of diabetes) may also play a part in high morning readings.

■ When you dress, choose clothes and footwear that do not bind or restrict circulation. Socks should not cause marks on your legs, and knee-high hose should be avoided. Socks should be made of a breathable fabric, and free from bumps, holes, and irritating threads that could cause undesirable pressure on the skin or bony prominences.

■ Pick shoes that are supportive and provide room for your toes to fit naturally, not pinched or bunched up. Good shoes are worth the money. Have your feet properly fitted to know your actual size. If you need to stand all day, visit a podiatrist or pedorthist who can help you choose shoes with adequate support or custom insoles.

■ Now that you're bathed and dressed, take your morning medication as directed, and note that you have taken it in your diary or logbook. Timing is very important with diabetes medications, as most must be coordinated with food. Consult with your pharmacist or health care provider to make sure you understand the right times to take your medications.

THE MOST IMPORTANT MEAL OF THE DAY

Breakfast isn't referred to as the most important meal of the day for no reason. Starting your day with a healthy meal can help kickstart your metabolism and make it easier to avoid glucose swings later. So eat your breakfast! If you don't like to cook, or need something simple, prepare a simple breakfast such as some of the following:

■ Toast with a slice of lean sandwich meat or low-fat cheese + 4 ounces of fruit juice

■ Unsweetened cereal with low-fat milk + 1 small piece of fruit

■ 8 ounces of low-fat yogurt with 1/4 cup of a high-fiber cereal mixed in

■ 8-ounce fruit smoothie (blended low-fat yogurt, ice, and fresh fruit)

■ Don't skip breakfast! Eat your prescribed meal plan. Many people underestimate the importance of breakfast, but any registered dietitian (RD) will tell you that you can't lose weight and control your glucose levels without breakfast.

- Don't forget to drink some liquids, at least 8 ounces. Start the day well hydrated. Check with your doctor about your caffeine intake and sweeten your tea or coffee with an artificial sweetener, not sugar.

- Brush your teeth. You should take special care of your teeth, as people with diabetes have a higher incidence of gum disease. This can happen at any age, so make sure you perform good oral hygiene morning and night.

- If you have time, perform morning exercises. Recommendations are to exercise 20–30 minutes each day, 5 days a week. If you don't have time in the morning, determine when you will exercise later in the day, and make the necessary arrangements.

- If you take insulin or an oral med than can lead to a low blood glucose reaction, make sure you have a hypoglycemia treatment (glucose tablets, glucose gels, juice, etc.) to take with you out the door, or to be near you in the home.

- Make sure you have regular identification, medical cards, and medical identification before leaving home.

- Take your diabetes supplies with you when you leave (medications, meter, strips, pump supplies, etc.). A small travel pack or cosmetic bag can make things easier. Cool packs are inexpensive and can help keep things at the proper temperature if needed.

- Spread some morning cheer to your family or fellow commuters. Diabetes is a disease that affects the entire family; remember to show support back to those who support you. Shared smiles are worth their weight in gold.

MORE RESOURCES TO EXPLORE

BOOKS

The Diabetes Dictionary. American Diabetes Association; Alexandria, VA, 2007.

(continued)

BOOKS *(continued)*

American Diabetes Association Complete Guide to Diabetes, 4th edition. American Diabetes Association; Alexandria, VA, 2005.

Caring for the Diabetic Soul, by Neil Friedman. American Diabetes Association and; Alexandria, VA, 1997.

365 Daily Meditations for People with Diabetes, by Cathy Feste. American Diabetes Association; Alexandria, VA, 2004.

WEBSITES

National Diabetes
Clearinghouse . . . . HTTP://DIABETES.NIDDK.NIH.
GOV/DM/PUBS/DICTIONARY/
This is the online Diabetes Dictionary of the National Diabetes Information Clearinghouse (NDIC), a division of the NIH. In addition to the dictionary, this website offers a wealth of information on a variety of diabetes subjects.

12

How to end the day

For most people, the evening hours of the day are a time to relax and enjoy time with family at home. A typical routine might be to come home, eat supper, walk the dog, watch some television, have a snack, and go to bed. So does having diabetes need to change your evening routine? It shouldn't. With a little knowledge of how food, activity, and medications affect your blood glucose, you should be able to manage your diabetes control, whether in your daytime or nighttime routine. There are, however, some things to consider. Common issues in the evening include snacking, medications, and safe nighttime blood glucose readings.

NIGHTTIME SNACKING

Depending on the type of diabetes you have and your diabetes control, your prescribed meal plan may or may not include a nighttime snack. Individuals with type 2 diabetes may not require a bedtime snack, especially if their meal plan is focused on weight loss and they are not taking medications that could lead to hypoglycemia. Consult with your RD to find out whether you should have a snack or not. The snacking urge sometimes results from not eating enough during the day or eating irregularly. Curb your desire to snack by eating your prescribed meals during the day. If your appetite persists, or you are experiencing undesirable weight loss, you need an adjustment in your meal plan.

Don't forget that snacking is eating. If you have been given a calorie or carbohydrate limit to follow, your snacks need to be counted in your plan. Some meal plans may allow 15–30 grams of carbohydrate for an evening snack. Choose the right carbohydrate amount, but don't forget about fat. Eating high-fat choices late in the day may cause high blood glucose readings during the night (leading to more trips to the bathroom in the middle of the night) and perhaps persistent high glucose readings the next morning.

If your meal plan includes an evening snack, consider some of the following lower-fat choices:

- Whole-grain cereal with skim milk
- Fat-free popcorn
- Fresh vegetables with a no-fat salad dressing dip
- Whole-grain crackers with low-fat cheese
- Nonfat yogurt with fresh fruit

There are some food choices that can be eaten in small quantities that don't need to be counted; these foods are often referred to as "free foods" and contain less than 5 grams of carbohydrate and 20 calories per serving. Some free foods include Jell-O and popsicles made with artificial sweeteners, one piece of hard candy, or one cup of plain popcorn. Talk with your RD for more free food suggestions.

HYPOGLYCEMIA FEARS AT NIGHT

If you have experienced a moderate or severe hypoglycemia (low blood glucose) reaction, you may be scared it could happen again. This fear particularly grows in the evening hours. People who take insulin often fear having hypoglycemia while they're asleep and "not waking up" to treat it, especially if they live alone. Don't worry; you do not have to fear hypoglycemia. Instead, with proper planning and management, you should be able to avoid a problem with hypoglycemia at night. Consider these tips:

- Check your blood glucose levels before you go to bed to catch problems before they happen.
- Follow your meal plan during the day.
- If your meal plan calls for an evening snack, eat only the specified amount. Eating more food than recommended

to "protect you" from having a low may backfire and cause more swings to occur with your blood glucose control.

- Talk with your health care provider about any fears you have about hypoglycemia.
- Be prepared. Have hypoglycemia treatments (juice box, can of soda, glucose tablets, packaged crackers, animal crackers, etc.) at the bedside ready to go. If needed, put the items in a zip-top plastic bag and label "For Hypoglycemia Only" so other family members won't be tempted to steal your treatment for a little snack themselves! Inform all household members of where the treatment is, in case you need help. Check this supply periodically to make sure the food is still fresh and appealing.
- Place a bell by the bed if you feel you may need help from someone within the home.
- Keep a glucagon emergency kit in the home, and make sure household members know where it is and how to use it.
- Have a phone at your bedside table if you live alone.
- If you experience nighttime hypoglycemia on several occasions, talk with your health care provider about this trend. It may be a sign you need to change your medication or treatment plan.

TIMING YOUR MEDICATION

Diabetes medications have changed over the years. Traditionally, medications were taken only at mealtimes. However, due to the expanding variety of diabetes medications, your medication may need to be taken at differing times, including bedtime. If your medication has been prescribed at bedtime, ask your health care team questions: Should you eat a snack? What time does your health care provider assume is bedtime? What if you work night shifts?

For example, let's say a diabetes medication last 12 hours. Your doctor has prescribed you to take it "morning and night." You may interpret this as before breakfast, when you rise, and at bedtime, when you go to sleep. However, this may only be 6–8 hours apart, rather than the intended 12-hour coverage time of the medication.

If the timing is not right, it's likely the blood glucose levels will not be right either.

BLOOD GLUCOSE TESTING

If your health care team suggests you check your blood glucose, ask whether you should check before bed. This may be helpful for a couple of reasons. If you take evening diabetes medication, you can check your glucose levels before you take the medication. If you are experiencing high blood glucose readings when you rise in the morning, checking your glucose before bed and in the middle of the night can give you valuable information. There are some recognized conditions associated with dips and rises in the evening, including the Somogyi effect (high glucose that follows a low during the night hours) and the dawn phenomenon (a change in hormone levels that causes blood glucose levels to rise on its own).

TURNING IN

Before turning out the light:

- Brush your teeth properly (individuals with diabetes have a higher risk of gum disease and mouth infections).
- If you bathe at night, read Thing to Know 22 on how to take a bath.
- Apply moisturizer on your skin if needed.
- Leave your glasses on your nightstand in case you need to get up.
- Turn on a nightlight in case you need to go to the bathroom in the dark, and clear a path from your bed to the toilet.
- Prepare for the next day to help the morning go smoother.
- Perform a relaxation measure such as reading, journaling, sewing, or crossword puzzles. Reducing stress can help reduce blood glucose levels.
- Tell the ones you live with that you love them, and thank them for any support they have given you with your diabetes that day.
- Think positive thoughts about the day that has passed and the new day to come.

MORE RESOURCES TO EXPLORE

BOOK

Diabetes A to Z, 5th Edition. American Diabetes Association; Alexandria, VA, 2003.

13

How to take diabetes to work

WHAT SHOULD YOU TAKE TO WORK?

Everyone with diabetes should take:

- Water bottle
- Medical ID/emergency phone numbers
- Medications (if needed)

If your health care team recommends you check your glucose levels:

- A working blood glucose meter
- Lancet device
- Lancets
- Test strips
- Container to hold used lancets (such as an empty vitamin bottle or small approved sharps container)
- Cotton balls or tissue

If you take insulin or another medication that can cause hypoglycemia:

- Hypoglycemia treatments that store well (glucose tablets or glucose gels)
- Snack for stabilizing hypoglycemia or if working late

CAN YOU STILL EAT WITH YOUR FRIENDS IN THE CAFETERIA?

Yes, of course. If your cafeteria has a rotating menu, take a copy of the menu to your next visit with your RD, who can help you make healthy choices. Even if there are some items that are "not the best," you can learn to modify the portion size to make it work for you. Most cafeterias offer salad bars, diet soft drinks, artificial sweeteners, and low-fat salad dressings—these items are used by everyone and will not make you stand out in the crowd or feel labeled.

CAN YOU STILL GO OUT TO EAT AT LUNCH?

Yes. Once again, work with your RD. You do not have to brown bag all your meals. To be discreet, call ahead to the restaurant if you are unsure what they offer—ask what could be substituted or what options exist. When you get to the restaurant, you already have a plan and less anxiety. If you end up at a restaurant with limited choices, don't be afraid to add an item or two from home to your meal.

ARE YOU ALLOWED TO TEST YOUR BLOOD GLUCOSE AT WORK?

Yes, of course, though you may need to discuss with your employer where you can access a clean, well-lit area. Make sure you follow safe sharps disposal practices (see Thing to Know 43 on getting rid of lancets, syringes, and other sharp items). To ensure you always have a clean space to work with and to prevent drops of blood from contaminating surfaces, tuck a small square of plastic wrap or wax paper into your testing kit each day. These are disposable and can be tossed away after testing.

WHAT IF YOU HAVE A LOW BLOOD GLUCOSE AT WORK?

If you take insulin or another medication that can cause hypoglycemia, you run the risk of having a low at work. Low blood glucose levels occur most often when you delay meals or are physically working hard. Carry low blood glucose treatments with you or keep a few in your desk or locker at work. Check these supplies each day to make sure you have at least two treatments as well as two emergency snacks. Tell your peers at work that you have diabetes and educate them on what your symptoms are for hypoglycemia and what treatments work best for you. Well-meaning friends may mistake a low blood glucose as a sign of a stroke, and with good intentions, may overreact to the situation. By keeping everyone informed beforehand, you can avoid serious incidents.

WHAT IF YOU HAVE TO LEAVE AN IMPORTANT MEETING TO TAKE CARE OF YOUR DIABETES?

High blood glucose levels can lead to frequent trips to the bathroom, headaches, or fatigue. Low blood glucose levels can lead to disorientation, blurred speech, and possibly, unconsciousness, all of which can be embarrassing—or dangerous! Do your best to keep your blood glucose levels stable so that swings do not occur at home or work. If you do have to leave, politely excuse yourself without blaming your diabetes for it. If you grouch about your diabetes being at fault for minor inconveniences or work performance to others, they will soon begin to believe it too, which may alter their impression of you.

HOW WILL DIABETES AFFECT YOUR PERFORMANCE AT WORK?

Having diabetes does not mean your performance at work will change. People with diabetes work all types of jobs, from CEOs of multimillion-dollar companies to part-time baggers at the local grocery store. Most people with diabetes do not have any health or physical restrictions that limit their professional choices in a career (though there are some restrictions, especially related to the military and airline industries). Some individuals will need to tell their employers they have diabetes so that "reasonable accommo-

DIABETES AND YOUR RIGHTS

It's unfortunate, but people with diabetes do sometimes face discrimination. If you'd like to learn more about your rights and what you can do to help, visit www.diabetes.org and click on the link to the Government Affairs & Advocacy section. There you'll find information on current legislation, health insurance issues, and your rights at school or the workplace.

dations" could be made, including access to an area to test blood glucose levels or take medication, regular work schedules, or set break times. However, there are still instances when people with diabetes have problems with their employers. So know your rights and never use your diabetes as an excuse for poor performance.

IS DIABETES A DISABILITY?

Not outright. A determination of disability status is made on an individual case-by-case basis, and must be pursued by legal procedures.

DO LABOR LAWS PROTECT YOU BECAUSE YOU HAVE DIABETES?

Yes. The Americans with Disabilities Act is a federal law that prohibits discrimination against people with certain disabilities as well as chronic diseases. The U.S. Equal Employment Opportunity Commission (EEOC) can provide information on diabetes in the workplace as well as the Americans with Disabilities Act in detail.

Talk with your benefits coordinator at work about other federal and state laws, including the Family and Medical Leave Act (FMLA), which allows time to be taken for the employee's or the employee's family's health condition, including frequent doctor's appointments or short-term off-work time. The American Diabetes Association also can be of support—advocacy is an important focus of the organization, and there are people who can provide answers to questions as well. If you'd like to learn more, call 1-800-DIABETES or visit www.diabetes.org.

WHAT CAN YOU DO TO HAVE A PRODUCTIVE WORKDAY AND CONTROL YOUR DIABETES AT THE SAME TIME?

▪ Develop a routine if possible.
▪ Get a good night's sleep to start each day refreshed.
▪ Eat before you leave home so that you have fuel for when you get to work. Not eating until you get to the coffee cart at work or have a morning break may cause your blood glucose

levels to go low. It can also make you tired and irritable, which is never good for productivity.

■ If you work different shifts, tell your doctor so he or she can help you modify your medication and meal schedules for day-shift days and night-shirt days.

■ If you experience mandatory overtime, be prepared with extra testing supplies and snacks at work.

■ Be sure you bring all the items listed earlier in this section.

■ See how your job affects your blood glucose. Take a week and test periodically throughout your work shift to see if you experience any trends. Take this information to your health care provider to help do some preventative planning to avoid swings.

■ After a long shift, you may feel quite tired. Test your blood glucose before you get in a vehicle or use public transportation to make sure your blood glucose levels are stable.

■ Find someone you can educate and trust who works with you, to help out in an emergency, if needed.

■ Provide emergency contact numbers to your Human Resources department or supervisor.

■ Perform daily stress management—no one performs their best when under stress.

MORE RESOURCES TO EXPLORE

WEBSITES

American Diabetes Association . . . . . WWW.DIABETES.ORG
Once again, the website of the American Diabetes Association is a great place to find information on rights, discrimination, and advocacy.

U.S. Equal Employment
Opportunity Commission . . . . HTTP://EEOC.GOV/FACTS/DIABETES.HTML
This section of the U.S. Equal Employment Opportunity Commission website, titled Questions and Answers About Diabetes in the Workplace and the Americans with Disabilities Act (ADA), *offers an extensive amount of information on your rights in the workplace.*

How to exercise without spandex and a gym membership

A membership to a local fitness center is a great way to get exercise in a safe and social environment. However, not everyone has access to a gym, and many may feel reservations about being in a fitness facility with others. Fortunately, there are 25 simple ways you can get physically active without a gym membership or a fancy spandex outfit.

25 WAYS TO EXERCISE AWAY FROM THE GYM

1. Give up 30 minutes of surfing the web or talking on the cell phone every other day and use this time to move your body.

2. Dance or walk in place while you talk on your cell phone or listen to your MP3 player.

3. Exercise your pet; they need physical activity, too. Brush them several times a week for 15 minutes, changing hands halfway through. This will work your arms and please your pet.

4. Exercise with your children or grandchildren. Don't just send *them* outside to ride their bikes; join them for a 20-minute bike ride, basketball or soccer practice session, or simple game of tag.

5. When driving, park in the spot farthest from the door of your destination. When taking public transit, get off at an earlier bus/train stop and walk the rest of the way.

6. Take the stairs instead of the elevator regularly.

7. Instead of a 10-minute coffee break, walk the halls or stairwells at your office to keep circulation moving.

8. While on the phone, perform chair exercises. Some sample exercises include:

▌ Foot raises—raise your feet off the ground, hold for a few seconds, lower to ground, and then repeat.

▌ Point and flex your toes—stretch gently and repeat several times.

▌ March in place.

▌ For long conference calls, switch on your speakerphone and do some air boxing.

▌ Arm circles are another easy activity. Switch the phone receiver from one side to another as you work each arm, or get a comfortable telephone headset so you have more physical freedom while on the phone.

9. While on the computer, perform leg exercises. Sample exercises include:

▌ Point your toes and draw an imaginary circle. Repeat several times with each leg.

▌ Raise your feet up on the ball of your toes, then rock back to your heels. Repeat several times.

▌ Leg extensions—sit tall, extend one leg upwards to the level of your hip, hold a few seconds, and then lower. Repeat with each leg.

▌ Thigh squeezes—sit tall, place a water bottle, small pillow, or small towel between your knees, and then squeeze your legs together and hold. Repeat several times.

10. If you are homebound with a child or grandchild, dance around the room or do yoga together during the day. Find a community center that offers parent/child classes.

11. Shop for produce at the farmer's market or large retail center and walk the stalls or aisles.

12. If your neighborhood doesn't have safe areas to walk, sweep your floors, porch, and driveway with an old fashioned broom several times a week.

13. Wash and dry dishes by hand. Wash the floor with a string or sponge mop, and polish windows and glassware.

14. Take the long way around in stores, walking the entire perimeter before you begin looking for the items you're there to buy.

15. Start a flower or vegetable garden, tending to it several times a week.

16. Instead of always planning to "go out to eat" with friends or family, plan an outing with physical activity as the event, such as hiking, Frisbee, walking through a zoo or a museum, or park. For couples, try dance lessons or a night at the dance club instead of a restaurant date.

17. Use less email at work and walk to the person down the hall to discuss business.

18. Walk to your favorite neighborhood restaurant rather than taking a cab or driving.

19. Walk with your child to and from the bus stop.

20. If your child has band practice, chess club, or soccer practice, walk around the gym or practice field while you're waiting. Or start an exercise club at your church.

21. Turn off the television after 7 P.M. three nights a week. With the TV off, you will likely find time for things you often put off, like household chores or a little 20-minute exercise session.

22. Participate in a museum hop. A museum hop is an opportunity to visit your city's local museums in an "open house" venue. Sometimes admission is reduced, and sometimes it is free. Food or drinks are often served. Check your local paper in the weekend or arts section to see if a "hop" is planned for your area. Your local arts council may also have a calendar of events for you to acquire so you can plan ahead.

23. Get a city map and explore a new walking place once a week, such as a historical site, cemetery, or public garden.

24. Use less motorized lawn care equipment and use old-fashioned rakes, hoes, and shears to burn more calories.

25. Rent some different home exercise DVDs until you find one that you like. Schedule time to watch and follow it.

SOME TIPS FOR EXERCISE

First and foremost, dress appropriately:

- Wear comfortable clothes, ideally non-binding and made from light, moisture-wicking fabrics.
- Choose properly fitting athletic shoes and leave the flip-flops or sandals at home.
- If it is an outdoor activity, wear a hat.
- If you'll be in the sun for more than a few minutes, apply sunscreen.
- Have a pocket or wear a pouch that holds your medical and personal identification.
- Wear a reflective vest if you'll be outside in dim light.

Watch your blood glucose:

- Check your blood glucose before you begin an activity, after the activity, and several hours later to see how the activity affected your blood glucose. Write down your results to see if you have any notable problems or trends.
- Carry a low blood glucose treatment with you. Glucose tablets are lightweight and easy to stick in a pocket or small pouch. Carry more than you think you'll need, just in case.
- For adventure activities or for the serious athlete, speak with a CDE, check out some books from the American Diabetes Association, or get tips from the Diabetes Exercise and Sports Association (see More Resources to Explore at the end of this section).

EXERCISE CAUTIONS!

- If you have type 1 diabetes, do not exercise on a day when your blood glucose is already higher than 250 mg/dl (or has been increasing steadily all day) or if you have had a positive ketone test during the last 24 hours. You could make your blood glucose go higher by exercising, which could lead to more problems or even diabetic ketoacidosis (DKA).

- Keep hydrated—drink water before, every 15 minutes during, and after the activity. Try 8 ounces at a time.
- A snack during may be needed if the activity is strenuous or lasts longer than 45 minutes. Talk to your RD first to avoid unnecessary calories before adding snacks. Usually, 15–20 grams of carbohydrate will be all you need to keep blood glucose levels stable.
- Learn to calculate your resting heart rate (see sidebar).
- If you take insulin, it might be best to exercise about 30–60 minutes after a meal, rather than before. This can help you avoid hypoglycemia.
- Some individuals with type 1 diabetes may need to alter their basal insulin (injections or pump settings) or their carbohydrate intake during and after activities. Consult your health care professional.
- If you have high blood pressure, retinopathy, foot problems, or are pregnant, check with your health care professional before starting an exercise program. You may need to avoid some types of activities. A physical therapist or exercise physiologist may be asked to help design a special plan if you have multiple health problems.

Calculating Your Heart Rate

Resting heart rate (RHR) is how many times your heart beats each minute. You can figure this out yourself. The count should only be taken when you are lying down and rested (preferably first thing as you wake up in the morning). To calculate your RHR:

1. You'll need a watch with a second hand or other timing device with second counts.

2. Find your pulse:
   - The easiest place is the neck. Gently press your first two fingers under your jawbone below your ear until you feel the pulse.
   - The next best place is the wrist. Gently press your first two fingers over the inner wrist just below the ball of your thumb.

3. Count each beat you feel during a timed 1-minute period and write the number down.

4. For accuracy, repeat this process on different days to verify your typical RHR. Plus, practice makes perfect!

Ask your health care professional what your target heart rate should be.

- Stop any activity if you have shortness of breath, feel faint, or experience any type of pain.
- You should be able to talk normally during activity. If you cannot, or feel very breathless, slow down or rest to avoid overexertion.
- You do not need to sweat heavily to get the benefits of exercise.
- Do a brief warmup (not stretching) before the activity and gentle stretching after to keep your muscles in good shape.

MORE RESOURCES TO EXPLORE

BOOKS

The "I Hate to Exercise" Book for People with Diabetes, 2nd edition, by Charlotte Hayes. American Diabetes Association; Alexandria, VA, 2006.

WEBSITES

National Diabetes Information Clearinghouse . . . . HTTP://WWW.DIABETES.NIDDK.NIH.GOV/DM/PUBS/PHYSICAL_EZ/INDEX.HTM
Another page on the National Diabetes Information Clearinghouse website titled, What I Need to Know About Physical Activity and Diabetes.

Diabetes-Exercise and Sports Association . . . . WWW.DIABETES-EXERCISE.ORG
The website of the Diabetes-Exercise and Sports Association.

Weight-control Information Network . . WWW.WIN.NIDDK.NIH.GOV
This is the website for the Weight-control Information Network, an initiative of the NIH.

15

How to make time for exercise in your busy day

Sometimes the truth hurts—exercise *is* good for you and that's the bottom line. Taking care of your body comes with some responsibilities, which take time out of the day. It may also take a few weeks for your body to adjust to a new lifestyle. The time you put into body care will be rewarded with a longer, healthier life. Think of it this way; if your doctor prescribed you a medication that helped:

- Blood glucose control
- Heart attack and stroke prevention
- Blood pressure control
- Weight control
- Strength
- Endurance
- Stress management
- Sleep disorders
- Fatigue and mental alertness

...wouldn't you take it?

HOW MUCH EXERCISE DO YOU NEED?

Current recommendations are to exercise 30 minutes a session, 5 times a week. More than likely, you'll need to work up to this amount. Plus, everyday activities burn calories, too. Still, nothing works as well as a dedicated, 30-minute session of aerobic or resistance exercises.

WHAT EXERCISES SHOULD YOU DO?

There are three different types of activity. Include different types in your activity plans:

- ■ **Aerobic:** These increase your breathing and help your heart. Examples include walking, swimming, jogging, and biking.
- ■ **Strength:** These increase your muscle flexibility and strength. Examples include lifting weights, using resistance objects like exercise bands, and balancing activities.
- ■ **Flexibility:** These help keep your muscles in good condition. Examples include yoga, stretching, dancing, and different types of martial arts.

DON'T THINK YOU HAVE THE TIME?

> If the President of the United States has time to exercise, don't you?

Most people complain that they don't have the time to exercise in an already overbooked schedule. Well, even recent Presidents—who have a pretty tough schedule—have been seen golfing, swimming, and jogging. The Secret Service can't exercise for them; they still had to do it themselves. If the President of the United States has time to exercise, don't you?

Still, finding time to exercise can be a challenge. Following are 15 tips and tricks you can use to find the time to exercise.

1. **Stop listing excuses**. If it is important to you, it will get done. As with your other diabetes management tasks, consider the costs and benefits of how exercise. While the rewards might not feel immediate in the beginning, you will begin to notice them more and more if you stick with it.

2. **Bundle it.** Plan for exercise to coincide with another daily activity. For instance, walk on the treadmill or use a stationary bike while you watch the morning news. Staying on a schedule can make all the difference. It will become a habit faster.

3. **Get some "me time."** Wake up 20–30 minutes earlier to fit it in before getting the kids up, which may mean skipping the late movie in the evenings. Does watching the news or the late

movie really improve your health? Probably not. Skip the news and set the alarm a bit earlier.

4. **Start small.** Never exercised, or has it been a while? Pick at least two days a week you can fit in 10 minutes of exercise. Over a few weeks, add extra time and then days until you reach your goal. By adding a few minutes at a time, rather than all at once, it will be easier to work a new routine into a busy schedule.

5. **Got 10?** Break up the time into 10-minute segments if you can't find the full 30 minutes to get it done. This method can still prove beneficial to your body. Remember, half a loaf is better than none. While you may get more benefits with a longer session, any movement is beneficial.

6. **Give your body a break**. Use part of your break time at work to engage in physical movement. If you plan to exercise after work, don't go home first—go straight to the location of your exercise. Once you open the front door to your house, you'll be surrounded by distractions.

7. **Blue Mondays.** Pick days on the calendar that will work. If Mondays are tough, don't schedule exercise for those days. At the same time, stick with the days you do choose. Plan for these days by using reminders to yourself—sticky notes on your bathroom mirror; alarm clocks or cell phone alarms; reminders on your PDA. Waiting for the perfect day to "happen" will likely mean never.

8. **Protect your exercise time.** Don't forfeit it to schedule other events. When exercising, off with the cell phone, bluetooth, pagers, and other distractions. If you let interruptions occur, you will lose minutes.

9. **Change it up**. Choose an activity that is interesting—if you never liked swimming, don't buy a Speedo. Vary your activity to keep from getting bored. Or find different partners for different activities—walking with your neighbor Sheila on Saturday, and Tai-Chi with Roger on Tuesday nights. Being bored will cause minutes to seem like hours and will decrease your motivation.

10. **Be a cheerleader.** Give yourself a small reward when you perform an activity—checkmarks on a calendar, treating yourself

to a rental movie, etc. A reward system will help you stay focused.

11. **Use timers or tools to help you track your progress**. A pedometer is a great way to help you measure your success. Strive for 10,000 steps a day, which is equal to about 5 miles. Write down your numbers to plot your progress to this goal.

ClubPed

If you have a pedometer and a computer, and you're looking for some extra support, try ADA's online walking group, ClubPed, at www.diabetes.org. Once there, you can track your progress, get tips on walking and exercise, and learn from others who have done it before.

12. **"I have limitations."** Get a trained professional to make recommendations about what types of exercises you can do, rather than just saying "I've got bad knees, I can't do anything," and doing nothing. Physical therapists or certified personal trainers may be able to suggest practical activities within your abilities that you haven't thought of. In fact, the exercise may help some of your other health conditions as well, not just your diabetes.

13. **Explore neighborhood resources**. Find local churches, malls, or schools that have safe, indoor walking tracks. This will "climate proof" your 30-minute stroll. Walking only on pretty days is bound to lead to problems once the seasons change.

14. **There's no place like home.** Buy home exercise equipment to save more of your precious time. If it takes more than 15 minutes to get to a gym or track, you are probably going to lose interest. Pick equipment that is within your abilities and has a small footprint—that $2,000 metal monster that kicks your car out of the garage is probably not the best choice. Position your home exercise equipment in the center of one of the most used rooms in the house—the kitchen, the family room, or your bedroom. Equipment in the basement or garage gets forgotten. In a corner, that treadmill quickly becomes an expensive clothes or quilt rack. Don't let home décor rules keep you from your personal health goals.

15. Get a buddy. They can help be your nag as well as cheerleader to stay motivated. Pick a partner who is as motivated or more motivated than you. If you pick someone you have to coach as well, it could be a poor partnership. We all need to spend more time on our relationships. Exercising together shows you care about your partner and his or her health, too.

FINAL THOUGHT....

You've heard of value meals? Walking or engaging in activity with a friend or a family member adds value minutes to both of your lives.

MORE RESOURCES TO EXPLORE

BOOK

Diabetes A to Z, 5th edition. American Diabetes Association; Alexandria, VA, 2003.

WEBSITE

Centers for Disease Control . . . . WWW.CDC.GOV/DIABETES/
CONSUMER/BEACTIVE.HTM
This address leads to the Diabetes and Me: Be Active section of the Centers for Disease Control website.

MAKE WISE FOOD CHOICES

How to reassure yourself that food as you know it is not over

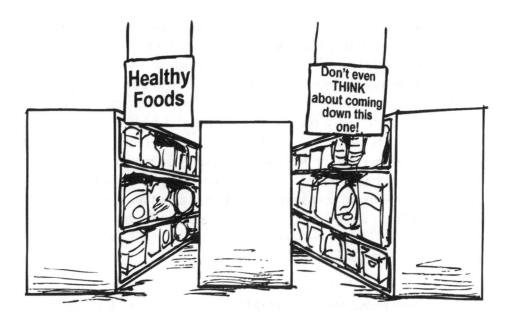

When you first learned you had diabetes, your first piece of meal-planning advice was probably a sarcastic, "If it tastes good, don't eat it." Whether it was a health care professional, family member, or friend, the advice was meant to be funny. Words, however, can have a lasting effect, and a phrase like that can negatively frame your view of meal planning for a lifetime. It also insinuates you will be giving up foods you like. Don't worry. Having diabetes means you will probably have to change the way you eat, but you won't have to abandon the foods you love.

WHY DO YOU EAT WHAT YOU EAT?

The food choices a person makes each day are made for a variety of reasons, including whether or not the food:

 ▌Looks good
 ▌Smells good
 ▌Tastes good
 ▌Digests well
 ▌Makes you feel full
 ▌Is socially accepted by friends and family
 ▌Provides a positive emotional response (comfort, pleasure, happiness, satisfaction)

It took many years for you to learn about foods and to decide what foods you like and what foods you'd rather sneak to the dog under the table. It will also take time to learn how to follow a new meal plan as well. Most of us choose a relatively narrow range of foods over the course of our lives. These limited choices may have been due to financial constraints, cultural and religious influences, family habits, or food availability. Whatever the cause, if you followed a somewhat limited diet in the past, you may be less likely to want to change your food choices now that you have diabetes. If you are willing to take some time to learn about food, you will discover that a diabetes meal plan offers variety and choices.

WHERE TO START

The best way to learn about a diabetes meal plan is from a nutrition expert—a registered dietitian (RD). The best way to follow any new way of eating is to make changes slowly, and don't let go of all your personal choices.

When you work with a RD or your health care team, you'll find that there are a lot of meal planning options, including the exchange/choices list, the point system, carbohydrate counting, or simple calorie counting. But no matter which method you decide to follow, the key to success will be portion control. If you don't already have some, spend a buck or two at the dollar store to purchase some measuring cups and spoons. These can help you learn how much of what goes on your plate.

Here are some other tips to help you follow a diabetes nutrition plan:

- Don't call it a diet.
- Make small changes on which you can build.
- Recognize that perfection is impossible.
- Set realistic goals.
- Ask your family to support you, not act as the food police. Ask them to share positive feedback, not negatives, with you during your transition.
- Adapt changes for the entire household.
- Forgive and forget errors and move on.
- Talk with a RD if your plan restricts your favorite foods.
- Experiment with new recipes/restaurants to make changes more appealing.
- Mark your progress (blood pressure, lipids, glucose, cholesterol, weight).
- Use reliable nutrition sources. Health care professionals, *not* hairdressers or neighbors, are the best sources of information.
- Avoid diet fads and unrealistic goals. Trying to lose 10 pounds in a week is just setting you up for failure.
- Ask for positive feedback and find your own reward system for your successes.
- Remember, food is a personal choice, and *the choice is up to you.*

MORE RESOURCES TO EXPLORE

BOOKS

The Diabetes Food and Nutrition Bible, by Hope Warshaw and Robyn Webb. American Diabetes Association; Alexandria, VA, 2001.

WEBSITES

American Dietetic Association . . . . WWW.EATRIGHT.ORG
This is the website of the American Dietetic Association. Here you can find all sorts of information on meal planning and healthy eating.

How to safely eat a baked potato and other adventures in carb counting

"GOOD" FOODS AND "BAD" FOODS

Learning about food can seem complicated, especially if you have never had to follow a special nutrition plan before. Meeting with an RD or taking a class will give you more knowledge about making proper food choices. One of the first things you will learn is that you're allowed a wide variety of foods. There is no such thing as a "good" list of foods or a "bad" list of foods. Instead, you will learn about the components of food and how they may affect your blood glucose and overall nutrition. With this knowledge, you will be able to make appropriate food choices.

WHERE TO START?

There are three main types of nutrients in the world of foods: carbohydrates, protein, and fats. Each type plays an important role in keeping your body going every day. A balanced meal plan will provide you with food choices from each of the three types of nutrients. Being able to identify what type of nutrient is in the foods you are eating is the best place to start learning about a diabetes meal plan.

During the day, you make many choices regarding food. Maybe you want to go out to lunch and see a tempting item on the menu; say, a stuffed baked potato. Is it safe to eat? With a little knowledge about foods, you will be able to make confident selections for each of your meals and those occasional snack attacks.

THE BASICS

Below are some lists that may help you identify what nutrient is in some of the different food groups.

WHAT FOODS CONTAIN THE NUTRIENT *PROTEIN*?

- Beef
- Chicken
- Pork
- Turkey
- Fish
- Game meat (venison, bison, rabbit, etc.)
- Tofu
- Eggs

WHAT FOODS CONTAIN THE NUTRIENT *CARBOHYDRATE*?

- Dairy products
- Fruit and fruit juices
- Vegetables
- Cereal and grain products (items made from wheat, rice, oats, and corn)
- Sugar and sweet products (honey, jam, jelly, syrups, candy, etc.)

WHAT FOODS CONTAIN THE NUTRIENT *FAT*?

- Oils
- Butter
- Margarine
- Mayonnaise
- Shortening
- Salad dressing
- Animal fats (meat fat, lard, drippings)

WHAT DO THE NUTRIENTS DO IN YOUR BODY?

After eating a meal, the different foods are broken down into their useable elements in your digestive tract. Your body keeps the useable parts, and the unusable parts are passed along the digestive tract for "disposal." Vitamins and minerals are used in different body functions, and the basic nutrients serve many purposes as well. Protein helps keep our bodies strong by building and maintaining the structural parts of the body. Carbohydrates primarily provide your body with energy (or fuel) to walk, talk, breathe, think, and perform other essential functions. Fats provide energy, too, as well as material needed to keep cells strong.

Technically, all of the nutrients provide energy, but carbohydrate is the primary source for our bodies. This is mostly because carbohydrates are a quick fuel that can be rapidly changed into the useable fuel glucose ("blood glucose") after eating. All of the foods, however, have an effect on your blood glucose levels and your overall nutritional health.

HOW MUCH OF EACH NUTRIENT DO YOU NEED EACH DAY?

This varies from person to person, based on your build, activity level, and health goals. No two people eat exactly the same. A tear-off sheet from the doctor just won't do. A written diabetes meal plan developed with the help of a RD is the absolute best way to determine how much carbohydrate, protein, and fat you should eat each day. This plan should be based on discussions you have with the RD that explain your lifestyle and your health goals. It is important to share what foods you like and dislike, listing any food allergies (if you have them) or food intolerances (foods that don't agree with you), cultural and religious food preferences, and lifestyle issues. This nutrition history is necessary to make a plan fit for you. Let your RD know how often you generally eat out, your snack habits, and your use of alcoholic beverages. With this information, the plan can be constructed in a way to make it easier for you to understand—and enjoy.

An individualized meal plan should have several objectives. It should:

1. Provide optimal nutrition (getting enough vitamins, minerals, and nutrients)
2. Help control blood glucose levels
3. Help control blood lipid (fat) levels
4. Help maintain or achieve a healthy body weight

5. Balance food timing with diabetes medications (if prescribed)

6. Make you feel satisfied with your meals

ONE SIZE DOES NOT FIT ALL

Fortunately, you and your health care team do not need to start from scratch when developing your meal plan. There are various types of diabetes meal plans to choose from. Some may be more general than others, but each is meant to help you carry out the nutrition prescription assigned by your diabetes care professional. The American Dietetic Association and the American Diabetes Association do not endorse one meal plan over another. However, people have successfully used the following popular meal plan methods:

- Food Pyramid
- Plate Method
- Exchange/Choice Lists
- Carbohydrate Counting
- Calorie Counting

In each method, you will learn how to choose healthy foods and eat proper portions.

WHAT ABOUT LOW-CARB MEAL PLANS?

The human digestive system is made up of several organs, each performing a special role in how we use food for fuel. The process of digesting food is a complicated and specialized process. Our body begins to digest food as soon as we take it into our mouths, when enzymes in our saliva begin to immediately start breaking down (metabolizing) some of our food, mostly carbohydrates. Because of this "jump start," carbohydrate foods will cause a faster rise in blood glucose levels than protein and fats, which require the lower parts of the digestive system to be broken down. Anyone with a blood glucose meter and a source of carbohydrate can attest that blood glucose levels will rise sometimes within minutes of eating carbohydrate food choices. This is a natural process in human beings, not just those with diabetes.

Unfortunately, because people with diabetes either don't make enough insulin or the insulin they do make doesn't work as well as it should, the normal rise in blood glucose is more pronounced and lasts longer. Considering that carbohydrate has such a pronounced effect on blood glucose levels, it would seem to make sense that eliminating them, or at least severely restricting them, would be a good idea, right? Well, not necessarily. Carbohydrate foods should not be removed from a diabetes meal plan. They simply offer too many vitamins, minerals, and other healthy nutrients that keep our bodies healthy. Some research has indicated that lowering total carbohydrate levels may help control glucose levels, but much more needs to be learned before this can be recommended. Your health care team will help you decide how much carbohydrate is right for your body's needs.

ARE SOME CARBOHYDRATES BETTER THAN OTHERS?

Carbohydrates can come packaged in different forms, such as a sugar, starch, or fiber. The form of the carbohydrate does make a difference in your blood glucose level. As you might expect, liquids (such as regular soda or fruit juice) are rapidly processed in our digestive system and tend to cause blood glucose levels to rise quickly. (Thank goodness they do, because they provide us with a quick solution to hypoglycemia.) However, this doesn't mean you have to completely eliminate juice from your meal plan. Learn what the proper portion size is, and work within those guidelines.

WHAT ABOUT THE GLYCEMIC INDEX?

The Glycemic Index (GI) is a method that has also been researched for use as a diabetes meal plan method. It may not be for everyone, because it requires investigating each individual food in detail. However, it has been demonstrated to help some individuals better control their blood glucoses after a meal. The GI method applies a "score" to all individual foods (not just the group) based on its ability to raise a person's blood glucose level when compared to a typical carbohydrate item—usually, a piece of white bread. Foods are scored on whether they have a low, moderate, or high GI level. These scores attempt to predict a food's effect on future blood glucose levels. Foods that have a high GI level are said to have a greater effect on blood glucose rises than those with a lower GI level. GI nutrition plans for people with diabetes generally recommend foods with low or lower GI index scores.

Another concept associated with GI is Glycemic Load (GL), an attempt to determine how the meals you eat, as opposed to just certain foods, will affect your blood glucose. The GL is derived using the GI of the food as well as the total carbohydrate in the food. Foods with a low GL score are said to have a lesser impact on blood glucose than high GL foods.

Carbohydrate type and content are not the only things that affect the GI and GL of a food. Cooking techniques, degree of ripeness, storage issues, variety of the product, as well as what other foods are eaten at the same time can all affect the impact on your blood glucose. For these reasons, individual responses to the same food will always vary slightly.

HOW DO I KNOW IF A CARBOHYDRATE FOOD IS "SAFE" FOR ME TO EAT?

To see how your body and your blood glucose respond to a food, do a little detective work on your own. If your friend "can't even touch a potato" because it launches her blood glucose sky high, don't just assume that you will have problems, too. For instance, your friend may not be considering portion sizes, which can have a huge effect on your blood glucose level. Most people do not realize that a standard serving of baked potato is only a 4-ounce spud. At restaurants and grocery stores, you are usually going to get a gigantic 12-ounce tuber. Dressing up your spud also contributes to its effect on your blood glucose—adding high-fat toppings such as butter, sour cream, cheese, and bacon will have an effect on your blood glucose, often delaying a high blood glucose and making it difficult to match medication to your glucose levels.

If you are still learning about food content, invest in a nutrient-counter book that contains carbohydrate information lists on common foods (see the More Resources to Explore box at the end of this chapter for examples). This inexpensive resource can help you make informed food choices in the future. Once you know what your overall daily and meal carbohydrate target amounts are, you can use the lists to help you map out a menu for today and the week ahead. Choose a reference book from a reliable resource, such as a health care organization, to get accurate and current information. Something from a popular magazine—whose sole purpose is to make money—may not be as trustworthy. New foods are frequently added, so pick up a revised edition every few years.

HOW TO TEST FOODS' EFFECT ON YOUR BLOOD GLUCOSE CONTROL

There is not a list anyone can give you of "perfect" foods for you, so, as mentioned above, you will need to do a little detective work. But how? Learning how certain foods and food patterns affect you will take time. Following is a plan of action you can take to conduct your own test. In the example, you would be looking at how a slice of cinnamon bread at breakfast affects your blood glucose.

Day 1 of test

1. Check your blood glucose before breakfast. If it is in an acceptable range (70–130 mg/dl), proceed. Record the result.
   ∎ If you are having hypoglycemia, stop the test and treat your hypoglycemia accordingly.
   ∎ If you are having hyperglycemia (blood glucose higher than 130 mg/dl), your blood glucose is already high, and testing a food may lead to inaccurate conclusions.
2. Eat your scheduled meal on time, and take your medications on time.
3. Choose foods from your meal plan in the proper portions (this example assumes that cinnamon bread is in your meal plan).
4. Check your blood glucose 1 hour after eating and record it in your log book.
5. Check your blood glucose 2 hours after eating and record it.
6. Check your blood glucose 3 hours after eating and record it.
7. After 3 hours, return to your normal management plan.

Before and after the test, try to eliminate any variables that may affect the results, such as physical activity, extra snacks, or medications you normally do not take.

Day 2 of test

Repeat all the steps from day one. Repeating the test helps to show whether or not the results recur, which is called validity testing. If the results are dramatically different, repeat the test again on another day.

Discuss the results, or your concerns about specific food choices, with your health care professional. You may want to compare certain choices with other foods. Change only one food choice at a time when you do the home testing. If you are struggling to find a day where your blood glucose levels are stable or provide consistent results, talk to your health care professional.

FOR THOSE WHO TAKE INSULIN

If you take insulin via a pump or are on an intensive multiple daily insulin regimen, you are probably familiar with advanced carbohydrate counting, and should already have an insulin-to-carbohydrate ratio and a sensitivity factor. If not, work with your health care team to develop one. Calculators and some specialized diabetes software programs can help with this task. Most insulin pumps also have features to help you calculate your insulin needs at meals. It is not uncommon to have different needs for different meals. If you are a pump user, work with your certified pump trainer and health care team to learn how to take advantage of these special pump features. Whether you take insulin by syringe or by a pump, using the method above to test the effect of certain foods on your blood glucose can be very helpful in determining your insulin needs.

MORE RESOURCES TO EXPLORE

BOOKS

The Complete Guide to Carbohydrate Counting, 2nd edition, by Hope Warshaw and Karmeen Kulkarni. American Diabetes Association; Alexandria, VA, 2004.

The Diabetes Carbohydrate and Fat Gram Guide, 3rd edition, by Lee Ann Holzmeister. American Diabetes Association; Alexandria, VA, 2007.

(continued)

BOOKS (continued)

Diabetes Meal Planning Made Easy, 3rd edition, by Hope Warshaw. American Diabetes Association; Alexandria, VA, 2006.

Pumping Insulin: Everything You Need for Success on a Smart Insulin Pump, 4th edition, by John Walsh and Ruth Roberts. Torrey Pines Press; San Diego, CA, 2006.

WEBSITES

Aemrican Dietetic Association — WWW.EATRIGHT.ORG/ADA/FILES/GLYCEMICINDEX.PDF

This is a link to a PDF document from the American Dietetic Association titled, Hot Topic: Glycemic Index, *which gives a good overview on the Glycemic Index.*

University of Sydney Glycemic Index Database . . . . WWW.GLYCEMICINDEX.COM

This is the website of the Official GI Newsletter.

USDA My Pyramid . . . . WWW.MYPYRAMID.GOV

This is the official website of the Food Pyramid Method.

Idaho Plate Method . . . . WWW.PLATEMETHOD.COM

This is the official website of "The Plate" Method.

USDA National Nutrient Database . . . . WWW.NAL.USDA.GOV/FNIC/FOODCOMP/SEARCH/

The USDA nutrient database provides free searches for nutrient compositions of foods.

How to start eating breakfast

With the hectic lifestyle most of us lead these days, meals are often eaten away from home or skipped outright in a rush to keep up with our daily agendas. The most commonly skipped meal is breakfast. Studies have shown that eating breakfast will help with attention and performance in children as well as adults. It can also help your blood glucose control. Eating regularly scheduled meals spaced throughout the day will help diabetes management by:

■ Controlling your appetite
■ Utilizing your medications more efficiently
■ Controlling blood glucose swings
■ Helping you interpret blood glucose information
■ Preventing hypoglycemia

5 STEPS TO EATING THE MOST IMPORTANT MEAL OF THE DAY

STEP 1—DEVELOP A SCHEDULE

Try to develop a realistic daily meal schedule YOU can stick to. Explain your habits and lifestyle choices to your health care professionals and build your plan around that.

■ Not hungry in the morning? If you routinely skip meals, you may have lost your physical cues for appetite. Try to eat three to five small meals regularly to see if your appetite will return.
■ Spreading calorie intake across three to five small meals can help prevent overeating and extra snacking, day or night.

Eating very late at night could be throwing off your normal appetite cues, as well as your blood glucose numbers.

▌Eating regularly will allow you to identify trends from one day to the next. This information is very valuable to discuss with your doctor. Don't settle for, "I can't control my blood glucose levels; they are always up and down, and there is nothing I can do." Eating regularly and being consistent will show if you do need treatment changes, or if there are further problems to explore.

▌CAUTION! If you work different shifts and cannot follow a routine, this information is important for your health care professionals to know. They will be able to work with you. If you don't communicate your lifestyle needs, controlling your blood glucose can become very challenging.

STEP 2—EAT SOMETHING, NO MATTER HOW SMALL, EVERY MORNING

If you have never eaten breakfast, start by eating at least one small item. Ideally, work your way up to the recommended meal plan established for you. You might start by simply eating a piece of toast. Then add a slice of low fat cheese for a source of protein.

> **TIP:** Read labels and compare brands. For instance, many breakfast cereals' marketing labels make the product look like a good choice, but read the label to be sure.

STEP 3—MAKE YOUR MORNING MEAL CONVENIENT

If you commute or run errands in the morning, choose a smoothie, health shake, or other beverage to sip on in a travel mug as you go.

▌Try a fruit smoothie made with ice, low-fat yogurt, and fresh fruit in a blender.

▌Try a milkshake, made with skim or soymilk, ice, and fruit.

▌Experiment with ready-to-go meal replacement beverages.

▌CAUTION! Beware of gourmet coffee beverages. A little squirt of this and a dollop of that can really add calories fast. Flavored coffees also often come with hidden sugars and calories. A 16-ounce Mocha Frappuccino from Starbucks contains 380 calories and 57 grams of carbs, which is almost like drinking a hamburger for breakfast.

STEP 4—TEST HOW SKIPPING BREAKFAST AFFECTS YOUR GLUCOSE

Skipping breakfast doesn't cause you problems? No symptoms? Do testing to prove your theory. Check your blood glucose every hour from the time you rise until lunch. If you find you have mid-morning hypoglycemia or glucose swings, you may have proof your body needs more fuel. Checking will either prove you were right or identify a fixable problem. Either way, you can't lose.

▮ Starting your day without fuel to sustain your body can lead to hypoglycemia, especially if you are active.

▮ Feelings of nausea or poor appetite may actually be signs of a low blood glucose; check to find out.

▮ "I'll just wait until I get to work." Your body depends on you to respond to signs of hunger and dropping or low blood glucose levels. Why put it off? Be prepared for hypoglycemia treatments at all times whenever you leave the house. Better yet—prevent it by taking a minute or two to eat.

▮ **CAUTION**! Getting behind the wheel of a car or leaving home when you feel yourself going low could risk your life and the lives of others. Check and stabilize your blood glucose before driving and carry low blood glucose treatments.

STEP 5—MAKE SURE YOU ARE GETTING THE MOST OUT OF YOUR MEDICATION

If you take medication in the morning, it might not be doing as much as it could if you don't balance the medication with food. Medication management means taking the right amount of medication at the right times and circumstances.

▮ An imbalance may mean your medications will not work as they were prescribed.

▮ Know whether your medication should be taken with or without food.

▮ **CAUTION**! At your next visit to the pharmacist, find out what to do if you miss a meal (i.e., should you still take your medication or not). If you take a medication that can cause low blood glucose, ALWAYS carry treatment with you.

MORE RESOURCES TO EXPLORE

BOOKS

The Diabetes Food and Nutrition Bible, by Hope Warshaw and Robyn Webb. American Diabetes Association; Alexandria, VA, 2001.

WEBSITES

Dairy Council of California. . . . . WWW.DAIRYCOUNCILOFCA.ORG
This is the website for the Dairy Council of California, which contains a section, "Good Nutrition: The first step to getting kids ready to learn," that deals with the importance of breakfast.

National Highway Traffic and
Safety Administration . . . . WWW.NHTSA.DOT.GOV/PEOPLE/INJURY/
OLDDRIVE/DIABETES%20WEB/
This web page, Driving When You Have Diabetes, was put together by the National Highway Traffic and Safety Administration in cooperation with the American Diabetes Association.

How to prepare a healthy lunch

No matter what your preference for lunch (brown bagging, drive thru, or restaurant dining), you need to make time to refuel your body. Your body prefers to have fuel spread throughout the day, especially during the active hours of the day. Some people make their midday meal their largest meal, while others make it a quick snack. Whatever the size, it is important to provide your body with the nourishment it needs to keep you feeling energetic through the rest of the day.

Having diabetes makes it harder to maintain your fuel levels. You need to balance the energy you are using throughout the day with food and medications (if taken). Several diabetes medications hit their peak activity in the body 4–6 hours after being taken in the morning. If you take one of these medications, you should strictly adhere to your meal schedule. It may take a bit more planning, but you can find appropriate food choices at home or away for your mid-day meal.

THE BROWN BAG

Tips for keeping your brown-bag lunch healthy:

- Carry reusable ice packs or freeze a water bottle or juice box to keep your foods cool. (If you carry a juice box, look for 100% juice or artificially sweetened products.)
- Carry your food in approved reusable containers—that empty cottage cheese container has likely not been

approved for reuse. Problems resulting from using non-approved containers include:

- Leaking/sealing problems
- Sanitizing problems
- Melting in the microwave
- Off flavors and odors
- Cross contamination

- Wash out your lunch containers daily.
- Pack a small container of hand sanitizer in your lunch bag to help you clean up before eating.
- Help save the environment. Use reusable containers rather than plastic bags and wraps to package foods. If you choose frozen entrees (these can be very convenient to pop in the microwave at work), recycle the trays.
- Portion foods yourself based on your nutrition plan using regular-sized food packages. Convenient, "single-serving" packets are usually more expensive and may not be the portion you need. Check the label before buying—if your convenience food doesn't have the portion you need or want, it may not be worth the extra money.

FOUR BROWN-BAG LUNCH IDEAS

1. Turkey sandwich on whole-wheat bread with lettuce and tomato; pretzels; whole piece of fruit; carrot sticks; and a beverage (preferably a non-caloric one, such as tea or water).
2. Ham and low-fat cheese wrapped in a tortilla or pita bread with spicy mustard; snow peas and red pepper strips; and low-fat yogurt topped with raisins.
3. Frozen, low-calorie prepared entree.
4. Large vegetable salad with diced low-fat cheese, chicken, and light dressing.

FAST FOOD DRIVE-THRU

Tips for keeping your drive-thru lunch healthy:

- Buy the kid's meal for smaller portions—it may also save you money. Many kid's meals now offer an optional fruit or vegetable side instead of French fries. Ask what your options are. Besides, you might get a fun toy for your desk at the office.

■ Research the nutrition information for your restaurant on the Internet, in books, or even on the wall of the restaurant. You may be surprised to see some of the items marketed as "grilled" may still have a lot of fat. Lesson to learn—choose items based on the nutrition labeling information rather than the title of the item. This can be a rude awakening, so be prepared.

■ Supplement your lunch with items from home. If you are a dashboard diner, carry a piece of fruit in your car to swap out with a poor fast food selection. Granola bars, dried fruit in zip-top bags, small bags of baked chips, or pretzels all have good shelf life and can give you options for side-orders. Be sure to clean out the car each night.

■ Choose lower-calorie side items such as side salads, fruit cups, or baked chips.

■ "Hold the cheese." Most cheese at fast-food restaurants contains a lot of fat and, in some cases, can add more than 100 calories to your sandwich. Sauces such as mayo, tartar sauce, and special sauces can add fat calories as well as carbohydrate. Choose sandwich toppings that are low in fat and calories, such as onions, vegetables, hot peppers, pickles, and mustard. Without the goo of the melty cheese substance, the sandwich won't be as likely to stick to the wrapper either, an extra benefit.

FOUR DRIVE-THRU LUNCH IDEAS

1. Child-size burger (hamburger, not cheeseburger) meal with a diet drink.
2. Sub-style sandwich with lean meat, lettuce, tomato, onion, hot peppers, and mustard; a side of baked chips or pretzels (small bag); and diet drink or water.
3. Grilled meat sandwich; side salad with diet dressing; and skim milk.
4. Bowl of soup or chili with side salad; crackers; and diet drink.

THE RESTAURANT

Tips for keeping your restaurant meal healthy:

■ Check online or call ahead and ask about menu choices in advance so you can be prepared.

■ If you take medications at meals, ask for the "express lunch" to avoid delays and get faster service. If you need to take the medication with your food, wait to take your medication until you actually SEE the food in front of you. Service can be unpredictable—it would be your luck that the restaurant is short-staffed and running behind the day you're there. If there is a delay and you feel you may risk a low blood glucose, ask for a cup of soup or a small salad to nibble on while you wait.

■ Ask if they will substitute a side salad or double portions of vegetables in place of large servings of starches or fried items. Remember YOU are paying THEM. You are not being a pain; just be polite and see what can be worked out.

■ Scan the menu for lighter side options or senior-meals. Don't be afraid to ask questions. Some "light" items may be lower in fat, but still considerably high in carbohydrate. They should have nutrition information available if they are making claims to it being "light" or "healthy."

■ Unless you're suffering a low glucose, skip the free chips, bread, rolls, or peanuts served as munchies on the table while you wait. They will add extra calories and may cause your blood glucose to have two separate "rises" from eating "twice."

FOUR RESTAURANT LUNCH IDEAS:

1. Choose a hearty vegetable plate or soup and salad option.
2. Grilled meat or seafood garden salad with diet dressing.
3. Baked or broiled meat or fish (4–5 ounces) served with two vegetable side dishes.
4. Stir-fry with vegetables with steamed rice and easy on the sauce.

MORE RESOURCES TO EXPLORE

BOOKS

The Healthy Lunchbox, by Marie McClendon and Cristy Shauck. American Diabetes Association; Alexandria, VA, 2005.

American Diabetes Association Guide to Healthy Restaurant Eating, 4th edition, by Hope Warshaw. American Diabetes Association; Alexandria, VA, 2009.

WEBSITES

USDA Food Safety and Inspection Services. . WWW.FSIS.USDA.GOV
This website is maintained by the U.S. Department of Agriculture, Food Safety and Inspection Services. Check out the section, Keeping Lunch Bags Safe.

HOW TO ACCURATELY WEIGH YOURSELF

▊ Weigh yourself at the same time every day, as fluid shifts throughout the day can cause your weight to fluctuate.

▊ Place your scale on a hard, flat, stable surface.

▊ Balance your scale before stepping on it. If you have an old-fashioned scale, use the little wheel on the back to make sure the indicator is idle at "0." Digital scales may have a button to "clear" or set to zero "0." Check your product guide for details.

YOUR WEIGHT 25¢
DESIRABLE WEIGHT $5

▊ Empty your bladder.

▊ Put on your birthday suit.

▊ Stand with both feet within the scale's boundaries.

▊ Be still.

▊ Look down and read the result.

HOW OFTEN SHOULD YOU WEIGH YOURSELF?

How often you weigh yourself is a matter of personal preference. On one hand, studies have shown that weighing yourself every day can motivate you to keep your weight under control. On the other hand, because your weight can be influenced by things like fluid retention and other factors, your day-to-day readings may not reflect how much body fat you have actually lost. Stepping on the scale after diligently following your meal plan and exercise regimen only to find you have gained two pounds can be very disheartening! Still, keeping track of your progress is never a bad thing, so weigh yourself often and just keep in mind that changes will occur from day to day.

BENEFITS OF WEIGHT LOSS

- Improved energy levels
- Positive self-image
- More clothes choices
- Better glucose numbers
- Better blood pressure readings
- Decreased risk of heart attack and stroke
- Less back pain
- Less foot pain
- Less leg pain
- Less knee pain
- Less medication (in most cases)
- More time on earth with your spouse/kids/grandkids/dog/cat/people who love you

IDENTIFYING WEIGHT-LOSS SCAMS

The vast majority of people in the United States would like to lose at least a little weight. With a market like that, it's no surprise that enterprising individuals have moved in to take advantage. While there are some excellent programs based on sound scientific evidence available, they are greatly outnumbered by programs filled with empty promises and flat-out wrong information. Generally, it's a weight-loss scam if:

- It sounds too good to be true. Except in very dramatic cases, losing 20 pounds in a week is unrealistic and usually related to fluid shifts rather than solid body weight change.
- It claims "you'll never crave [insert favorite food here] again"
- It requires you to buy expensive specialty foods or supplements for a long-term solution
- There are no references or resources cited on the program materials
- "Scientific" claims are not backed up by material published in approved medical journals (check with a reference librarian or medical librarian, found at a local hospital or medical school, to learn about credible health journals)
- A celebrity claims it is "perfect for everyone"
- It encourages skipping meals
- It describes certain types of food as "bad" or makes statements that conflict with those from the USDA or other recognized health organizations
- It states "you don't have to exercise" to lose weight
- It states it can "focus fat burning" in one specific body area (stomach, thighs, buttocks)
- It severely limits food choices (no "white foods," no "dairy," etc.)

SAFE WEIGHT-LOSS PLANS

If so many weight-loss programs are not to be trusted, how do you spot a valid program for losing weight healthily? Generally, a weight plan is safe and reliable if it:

- Encourages losing approximately 1–2 pounds a week
- Teaches you about proper food portions
- Teaches you what calories are and how much you need each day
- Provides education on nutrition for a lifetime, not just for a quick ten pounds
- Provides the credentials of the instructor (ideally a RD)
- Provides reliable support, not just a pamphlet

- You monitor other aspects of your health (blood pressure, blood glucose, etc.), not just weight
- Includes your favorite foods
- Is based on regular grocery store items
- Teaches you how to read a food label
- Provides a wide variety of foods to choose from
- Includes physical activity as part of the weight-loss strategy
- Provides information on "relapse" prevention as well as realistic goal setting
- Includes more than just one visit to a counselor or professional

MORE RESOURCES TO EXPLORE

BOOKS

101 Weight Loss Tips for Controlling and Preventing Diabetes, by Anne Daly, Linda Delehanty, and Judith Wylie-Rosett. American Diabetes Association; Alexandria, VA, 2002.

The Complete Weight Loss Workbook, 2nd edition, by Judith Wylie-Rosett. American Diabetes Association; Alexandria, VA, 2007.

WEBSITES

American Dietetic Association . . . . WWW.EATRIGHT.ORG
The website of the American Dietetic Association has a wealth of information. There you can find the nutrition fact sheet, "Popular Diets Reviewed," as well as the "Good Nutrition Reading List." They also have a RD finder that can help you locate RDs in your area.

CHAPTER 5
DO YOUR DAILY ACTIVITIES

21. What to take with you when you walk the dog

22. How to take a nice bath

23. How to take care of your feet and ten toes

24. What to do when you forget your medications

25. How to make time for your health

What to take with you when you walk the dog

When you have diabetes, everything seems to require thinking and decision-making, even taking Spot for a walk. This is because diabetes is not something you can just leave on the shelf at home. It goes with you everywhere. Activity and food affect your blood glucose levels, so actions inside and outside the home play a part of your control. Changes in your routine can cause your blood glucose to rise or fall. In addition, unexpected situations, such as getting stuck in traffic, meal delays at a restaurant, or extra hours at work, can pop up. It is always better to take a few minutes to prepare for what you know is going to happen when you walk out the door, as well as to prepare for the unexpected.

TIPS FOR STAYING PREPARED

Carry ID. Always wear some form of medical ID when you leave your home. This will do the talking if you're in an unexpected emergency and cannot speak for yourself. If you need emergency care, having others know you have diabetes can affect treatment decisions and could contribute to the success of the interventions. Many retailers offer medical ID cards, bracelets, necklaces, and watch charms. Look in the back of any health-related magazine to find advertisements, or ask at your local pharmacy. If you'd like something nice, some jewelry stores can order more upscale forms of ID.

Set speed dials. Pre-program your mobile phones with emergency numbers, such as 911 and your emergency contacts.

Cover those toes. Even if you plan to simply step out to grab the mail, don't forget to put on some footwear. Going barefoot is not advised, as there can be hidden dangers even within your own manicured green lawn. You need to take special precautions with your feet, and the most important rule is to prevent an injury before it happens, so keep a pair of yard shoes by the door to help remind you. The shoes should cover your entire foot, so no flip-flops—they offer little protection or support.

Can you hear me now? If you plan to be in the yard for some time, let someone know where you are, what you are doing, and for how long. If you planned a stopping point, stick to it. Pushing yourself to do extra work may lead to a hypoglycemic event. Inexpensive walkie-talkies can be used as a means to communicate if necessary.

U need SPF. Being outside also will require protection from the sun—people with diabetes tend to have drier skin and may sunburn more easily. Wear at least SPF 15 or higher sunscreen, and wear protective hats and clothing to prevent burns. Have a source of fluid to stay hydrated.

Be like a teen. Stick the mobile phone in your pocket if you will be alone on a long neighborhood walk, or walk in the park, or stroll in the country. Teens never leave home without a mobile phone; neither should you.

Know your turf. If you walk the same paths to work, school, or the gym, take note of available public phones, stores, or other areas where people might be available to help if necessary. Get to know some of the folks in the neighborhood as an extra security measure.

Look at the clock. Plan events that involve physical activity after a meal rather than before to prevent low blood glucose reactions. Activity lowers blood glucose, so use this tactic to help lower glucose levels following a meal.

Guardian angels. Inform someone of your whereabouts if you are doing something unusual or out of your usual routine. A quick call can reassure a coworker or family member. They worry.

Driving under the limit. If you take insulin or a medication that can lead to hypoglycemia, you should check your blood glucose before driving a car. Do not drive or leave if your blood glucose appears to be dropping to unsafe levels or you are already sensing a possible low symptom. Don't leave home until your blood glucose is stabilized. This is especially important when attempting drives longer than 30 minutes or a drive several hours after a meal.

Carry carbs. Finally, and most importantly: If you take insulin or an oral med that can cause hypoglycemia, always carry some form of low blood glucose treatment with you when you leave home. These are NOT snacks, so don't let your daughter (or your hungry belly) convince you otherwise. They are there to treat a medical condition. (See box Hypoglycemia: Symptoms and Treatment for more.)

HYPOGLYCEMIA: SYMPTOMS AND TREATMENTS

Hypoglycemia is the medical term for a low blood glucose, which is officially a glucose level lower than 70 mg/dl. This primarily affects those who take insulin or oral medications that can cause hypoglycemia (e.g., sulfonylureas).

COMMON SYMPTOMS OF HYPOGLYCEMIA

- Feeling weak
- Feeling shaky
- Feeling dizzy
- Feeling tired (frequent yawning, feeling down)
- Feeling hungry
- Mood changes
- Sweating
- Tingling of lips or hands
- Inability to think clearly or answer question

(continued)

TREATING HYPOGLYCEMIA

To treat a low blood glucose reaction (blood glucose <70mg/dl), eat 15 grams of quick-acting carbohydrate. Examples include:

- 1/2 cup (4 oz) fruit juice
- 1 cup (8 oz) milk
- 4–6 oz regular soda, sweetened sports drink, or other sugary beverage
- 1 tablespoon honey, corn syrup, or pancake syrup
- 2–3 glucose tablets (15 grams carbohydrate)
- 1 tube glucose gel (15 grams carbohydrate)
- 2–4 pieces of peppermint or other hard candy

A follow-up snack, consisting of 15–30 grams of a solid form of carbohydrate (crackers, cereal, etc.) may be needed to help maintain a blood glucose level after a reaction. Some situations when a snack may be called for include:

- Having a hypoglycemia reaction during a sport activity that is not yet over
- Having a hypoglycemia reaction while you are driving
- Having a hypoglycemia reaction when there are still several hours to go until you eat a meal
- Having a moderate level of hypoglycemia
- Being a young child or active adult

After treating, recheck your blood glucose an hour later to make sure your blood glucose has stabilized.

THINGS TO KEEP IN MIND

- If you get symptoms of a low blood glucose when you are away from home and you do not have a blood glucose meter with you, go ahead and TREAT it as if you KNOW you are low rather than guessing.
- Do not over-treat! A low blood glucose makes you feel very anxious and crummy, so it is very common to over-treat and wind up with high blood glucose levels later on. These types of swings will cause a

rotten day full of symptoms, but primarily a feeling of fatigue. Prevent over-treatment by creating in advance low blood glucose emergency kits with portion control (such as small juice boxes and select packages of crackers) in small zip-top plastic bags or lunch bags.

■ Anyone who takes insulin or oral meds that can cause hypoglycemia can get a low blood glucose reaction; it doesn't matter what form of diabetes you have. If you are having hypoglycemia multiple times a week or at certain times of the day or night, or have moderate to severe symptoms, talk to your physician or health care provider.

■ Be open with your friends, family, and neighbors. Take 15 minutes with them to educate them on your symptoms and your preferred treatment. Show them where you keep supplies.

MORE RESOURCES TO EXPLORE

BOOKS

Diabetes A to Z, What You Need to Know About Diabetes – Simply Put, 5th edition. American Diabetes Association; Alexandria, VA, 2003.

WEBSITES

National Institutes of Health. . . . . HTTP://DIABETES.NIDDK.NIH.GOV/DMA-Z.ASP
This website offers a free booklet, Prevent diabetes problems: Keep your feet and skin healthy (2008). This booklet can also be obtained by calling 1-800-860-8747.

MedIDs.com. . . . . WWW.MEDIDS.COM/FREE-ID.PHP
This website offers a free medical ID you can print off at home. Simply fill out the online form and print.

Children with Diabetes. . . . . WWW.CHILDRENWITHDIABETES.COM
Comprehensive directory of medical ID products, including gold, silver, sport, and children styles.

Paddock Labs. . . . . WWW.PADDOCKLABS.COM
Website for Paddock Labs, makers of the Glutose 15 hypoglycemia treatment product.

BD. . . . . WWW.BDDIABETES.COM
BD hypoglycemia treatment tablets and information about hypoglycemia. You can also call 1-888-BDCARES (1-888-232-2737).

22

How to take a nice bath

PROTECTING YOUR SKIN IS VITAL

Your skin is the largest organ of the body, providing protection 24 hours a day against the elements of the world. Unfortunately, recurring high blood glucose levels can damage your skin in several ways:

▌High blood glucose levels for long periods of time can damage your nerve cells, which perform the function of sensation, such as touch and sensitivity to temperature. This damage is called diabetic neuropathy. The result can be sharp or recurring pain or an absence of feeling in various parts of your body, primarily your fingers, hands, feet, and toes. Diabetic neuropathy is a risky condition, as it can damage your skin and the tissue underneath without you being aware of it. There are many stories about people unknowingly stepping on items that pierce or damage their foot, but then discovering only much later that they had suffered a violent

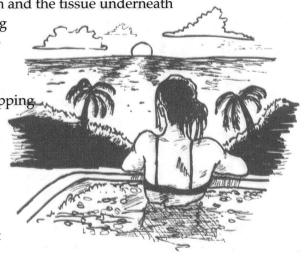

injury. Unfortunately, an untreated injury can rapidly escalate into a raging infection, which can have very serious consequences.

∎ High blood glucose levels also can cause dry skin. Too much glucose in the blood for long periods of time causes the body to try to get rid of the glucose by excreting the glucose through extra urine production. Loss of fluid can cause dry skin, which can lead to irritations, cracking, and possible infections. Further, nerve damage to the skin cells can also impair your ability to sweat, which normally works to keep your skin hydrated and supple.

∎ High blood glucose levels for extended periods will cause damage to your circulation. Poor circulation can lead to recurrent illnesses and infections as the body cannot defend itself as well. If left unchecked, the circulation can worsen further in your extremities, causing a condition known as peripheral vascular disease.

15 TIPS FOR SKIN-SAVING BATHING

Commit yourself to daily skin care. Here are some suggestions on how to take a nice bath in order to lower your risk of skin problems.

1. Make the bathroom a safe place to bathe.

∎ Keep towels, clothes, and magazines off the floor.

∎ Use a bathmat with non-skid backing to prevent falls. Don't just throw down a regular towel that can turn into a skateboard on a wet tile floor.

∎ Use a rubber mat or rubber sticks on the floor of the tub to give you firmer footing.

∎ If you have decreased mobility, purchase and properly install safety rails and bars. These are available at most local medical supply or hardware stores.

∎ Keep items in reach so you do not have to stretch or strain to reach the shampoo or soap.

∎ Keep your bathtub clean. Use appropriate products to keep out the ring, as well as extra germs. You can sanitize your tub with one part bleach to one part water solution weekly.

2. Take necessary items in with you, so you do not have to get up wet and possibly fall trying to retrieve your favorite robe and slippers.

3. Draw a warm bath, but not a hot bath. Some resources recommend no higher than 105 degrees, just a few degrees higher than body temperature. Hot water can worsen dry skin and could cause a burn. NEVER dip your foot into a tub to check the water temperature! You could cause a burn to your feet, a very hard place to heal. Use your elbow, wrist, or back of your hand to test the water. If you have diabetic neuropathy and decreased sensation, invest in a water thermometer to help you determine the water temperature. Children and baby supply stores often carry these water-tolerant floating thermometers. If you get lucky, you might find one in the shape of a duck at your local store so you don't have to bathe alone.

4. Open/close your bathroom doors or adjust your thermostat to prevent condensation from building up and causing slick surfaces.

5. Carefully step into the tub.

6. Use a mild moisturizing soap to wash yourself. Don't forget to wash your "corners," such as between your toes, the pits of your arms and knees, and your private areas. Use a soft washcloth to provide light friction on your skin.

7. While it may seem inviting to soak, staying in the water too long can further dry your skin. After washing, carefully step out of the tub, keeping at least one hand and one foot on sturdy surfaces while rising.

8. Pat yourself dry with a clean, soft towel. Do not rub. Dry the "corners" you just cleaned well. Skin under the breast, in the groin, or in other body folds is more likely to get fungal infections if the areas frequently stay moist.

9. Close your toilet lid, place your towel on top, and carefully sit down.

10. Look at your body one area at a time to inspect for skin problems such as reddening, dry or painful spots, new cuts or scrapes, blisters, calluses, or skin problems. Take extra time on your feet and toes. If you are able, ask a member of your health care team at your next appointment to teach you how to perform a monofila-

ment test on your feet. Periodically performing this test can help you assess the nerve function of your feet and toes.

11. Apply a gentle moisturizing lotion just after bathing to help lock in some moisture from the bath. Ask your doctor or health care provider what skin product they recommend. It is usually worth the money to buy a higher-quality lotion, as the lesser expensive ones may evaporate quickly, or worse, contain drying agents (alcohols and some other chemicals). Some products may contain vitamin E, which is a nutrient known to help skin condition. Do not apply lotion in between your toes or in the areas of your body where there are folds—this may promote bacterial or fungal growth. They love a warm, moist environment!

12. Wear all-cotton underwear, or at least a blend. Cotton fibers allow air movement, which helps your skin stay the right temperature. Newer fabrics that help wick moisture away and allow circulation are also showing up on the market. Discard any undergarments that cause visible impression lines or chafing. Women should have properly fitting bras, and can get a professional to help with fit at many department stores with lingerie agents.

13. Wear slippers or house-shoes that fit around your entire foot. They should have non-skid soles.

14. Frequently change towels.

15. Leave a nightlight on for visibility after you go to bed.

MORE RESOURCES TO EXPLORE

BOOKS

Diabetes A to Z, What You Need to Know About Diabetes – Simply Put, 5th edition. American Diabetes Association; Alexandria, VA, 2003.

101 Tips on Foot Care for People With Diabetes, 2nd edition, by Jesse H. Ahroni and Neil M. Scheffler. American Diabetes Association; Alexandria, VA, 2006.

WEBSITES

American Podiatric Medical Association . . . . WWW.APMA.ORG
  Website of the American Podiatric Medical Association. You can also get information by calling 1-800-FOOTCARE.

Neuropathy Association . . . . WWW.NEUROPATHY.ORG
  Website of the Neuropathy Association. More information is available by calling 212-692-0062.

National Institutes of Health. . . . . WWW.NIDDK.NIH.GOV
  Website of the NIDDK, a division of the NIH. Here you can find the brochure, "Take Care of Your Feet for a Lifetime, a Guide for People with Diabetes." You can also order the brochure by calling 1-800-860-8747.

National Institute of Arthritis and
  Musculoskeletal and Skin Disease. . . . . WWW.NIAMS.NIH.GOV
  Website of the National Institute of Arthritis and Musculoskeletal and Skin Disease (NIAMS), another division of the NIH. You can also call 1-877-226-4267 for more information.

PUBLICATIONS

Diabetes Skin Care (2007). Consumer Health Division, 3M, Nexcare, St. Paul, MN, http://solutions.3M.com, 1-888-3MHELPS, accessed July 2009.

Prevent diabetes problems: Keep your feet and skin healthy (2008) [free booklet]. (NIH Publication). National Institutes of Health, accessed July 2009 from http://www.diabetes.niddk.nih.gov/dm/pubs/complications_feet/index.htm, or 1-800-860-8747.

23

How to take care of your feet and ten toes

There is a saying in the horse industry: "No hoof, no horse." The same can be said of people. You may have been told that your hooves, or feet rather, demand special attention now that you have diabetes. You may have also heard of an unfortunate situation where an individual had lost a toe or limb through amputation due to complications related to diabetes. However, this does not mean everyone must suffer the same fate. If you "stay on your toes" with your diabetes management, you stand a better chance of keeping your own toes healthy.

Sometimes it is hard to correlate the readings on your hand-held blood glucose meter to the future health of your body, such as your ten toes. But you should make an effort to keep your blood glucose in a target range each day, as it can affect the circulation and the sensation in your toes. Without good care, damage to your extremities can occur and may not be reversible.

> "If you "stay on your toes" with your diabetes management, you stand a better chance of keeping your own toes healthy."

The good news is that an ounce of prevention now is worth pounds of cure later when it comes to your feet and toes. Feet are often neglected during the day as we pound them over all sorts of terrains, squash them into unsuitable shoes, and put all of our weight on the matrix of tiny bones that make up our foot structure. Considering what we put them through, you would think our bodies would have large bones and tough armor on our human feet. Instead, we have a more delicate structure, surrounded only by a layer of skin.

You have the primary responsibility of taking care of your feet each day—they are attached to YOU not your doctor. Your health care provider also must participate by checking your feet at every visit (take off them socks, even if they don't tell you to; you ask if they don't!) and monitoring your health status (glucose control, cholesterol control, blood pressure control, circulation, etc.). But you should perform foot checks daily.

15 STEPS TO GOOD FOOT CARE

Give your feet the respect they deserve, and perform the following steps to keep them in great shape.

1. **Take a long, hard look**. Each day, thoroughly inspect your feet. There is no greater act of prevention than awareness. Wear glasses or use a magnifying glass (some medical aid stores carry a device with a lens on the end of a long stick for better viewing) and use good light. Note any skin color, temperature, sensation, or integrity changes. Take a peek between each of your toes, especially in the folds, which is an often forgotten geographic place on your body.

2. **Perform daily care**. Wash your feet daily in warm (not hot) water, and use a soft cloth to clean between the toes. Use a pumice stone to gently rub on old calluses to help remove them over time. Foot massages can feel great and help the circulation, too.

3. **Protect them from the world.**

   ■ Do not share nail polish and nail tools with others—you may end up with fungal infection.
   ■ Guard against getting plantar warts, athletes foot, or other foot "cooties" at the pool by wearing water-shoes into the bathhouse or other wet areas.
   ■ Use nylon footies or your own socks when trying on shoes at the store.
   ■ ALWAYS wear shoes, indoors and out.

■ Protect any foot or toe injury well with the recommended dressings or bandages of your health care provider. If you aren't sure what your health care provider would do for a toe blister, ask. Chances are there may be more detail to it than you realize—antibiotic cream, bandages, pressure relief, etc.

■ Make sure your pedicurist follows all local health department rules.

■ Have shoes for all seasons: wet, dry, hot, or cold.

4. **Stick in your hand, not your foot, first.** Inspect every type of footwear (slippers included) with your hand before putting them on. Rover may have dropped by for a late night chew and damaged the rims or toes of your shoes or slippers, which could cause a friction blister later. Small items can easily drop into shoes in busy households: a paperclip, dry cleaning pin, pebbles, cat litter, you name it. Get rid of shoes that start to lose support and have developed areas of friction or discomfort.

5. **Sock it to them gently.** Wear properly fitting socks. Avoid socks that leave indentations or redden areas after wearing. Choose socks with breathable fibers to keep moisture down and air circulating. Do not wear socks that have been darned or that are holey—pitch them out.

6. **Knee-highs are kno-kno.** Women should avoid wearing knee-high stockings as these are usually very binding on the leg. Wear panty hose or quality trouser socks instead. It is important to keep the circulation going—it's what keeps YOU going.

7. **Fashion that fits.** Wear properly fitting shoes—fashion comes and goes, but your toes must endure. Purchase good quality shoes with support and comfort in mind. Get your feet properly measured by a shoe store expert who can advise you on what length and width you really need. You may not really be a size 6 1/2 Medium width, even if that's the size of those pretty brown pointy-toe shoes that would look just great with your new suit. If you find a store that usually carries your size or a brand that works well for you, ask the store clerk about special ordering.

They want your business and may be willing to do special orders.

8. **Breaking in is hard to do.** Break in new shoes slowly, only an hour at a time at home, before testing them out in the real world. Most stores will take back shoes if you discover they are not a good fit—as long as they do not show signs of wear. So don't plan to wear those shoes for the first time on a night out across town.

9. **A what?** A certified pedorthist is a person who has received special training in fitting people for shoes. If you are struggling with comfort even though you have tried expensive shoes recommended by friends or health care providers, seek out a local certified pedorthist to help you. You may need a simple insert or other shoe adjustment to make your shoes fit well. If you stand on your feet for long periods of time on hard surfaces, you may want to consult a pedorthist about a cushioning layer to prevent having leg/hip/back pain from prolonged standing. Add these people to your care team if needed.

10. **Just a trim, not a cut.** Ask your health care provider how to properly and safely trim your toenails. By doing regular trims, you can avoid having to do more difficult cutting as the nail can become thick and ragged. Use proper tools—not a pocketknife or worn-out clippers from years ago. Some individuals recommend trimming them after a shower or bath while the nail is still softer to avoid brittle tears and cracking. If you can no longer perform this function for yourself, ask to be referred to a podiatrist, not a pedicurist.

11. **A tiny little tool**. Ask to be taught how to use a home monofilament to help you evaluate sensations in your foot (all sides) and your toes (tips and tops, too!). Monofilaments are specially designed, tiny little plastic sticks that allow you to touch areas on your feet and toes

to see how well you feel the sensation. Don't get creative and design your own testing tool, you could cause injuries. Regularly using a monofilament after a bath or shower can help you identify sooner when a sensation problem (neuropathy) begins to develop. The faster a problem is discovered, the sooner the treatment can begin.

12. **Maintain a safe environment.** Do not apply petroleum jelly, creams, or lotions in-between your toes. This extra moisture can create an environment for foot problems to develop.

13. **The drug store is not a doctor's office.** Have warts, corns, toenail cracks, ingrown nails, calluses, and blisters inspected by a health care professional and treated as soon as they are discovered. Avoid the urge to self-treat; some over-the-counter products can cause further damage. Quick, do-it-yourself remedies may appear to save you money, but may cost you in the end.

14. **Will insurance pay for special shoes?** Special shoes may be necessary if you have significant structural issues with your feet such as bunions, hammertoes, arch problems, or pressure-related injuries. Check with your health care professional about seeing a shoe specialist, or podiatrist. Also check if you are eligible for insurance coverage. Medicare does allow some coverage, so check into it with your plan provider.

15. **Stay active!** Physical activity will help you keep the blood circulating and allow your body to help protect your feet from the inside out.

MORE RESOURCES TO EXPLORE

BOOKS

101 Tips on Foot Care for People With Diabetes, 2nd edition, by Jesse H. Ahroni and Neil M. Scheffler. American Diabetes Association; Alexandria, VA, 2006.

WEBSITES

American Diabetes Association. . . . . WWW.DIABETES..ORG/TYPE-2-DIABETES/FOOT-COMPLICATIONS.JSP
This section of the American Diabetes Association website deals specifically with complications of the foot.

American Podiatric Medical Association . . . WWW.APMA.ORG
Website of the American Podiatric Medical Association. You can get additional information by calling 1-800-FOOTCARE.

Pedorthic Footwear Association . . . . WWW.PEDORTHICS.ORG
Website of the Pedorthic Footwear Association. More information is available by calling 1-800-673-8447.

Neuropathy Association . . . . WWW.NEUROPATHY.ORG
Website of the Neuropathy Association. More information is available at 212-692-0062.

National Institutes of Health . . . . WWW.NIDDK.NIH.GOV
Website of the NIDDK, a division of the NIH. Here you can find the brochure, "Take Care of Your Feet for a Lifetime, a Guide for People with Diabetes." You can also order the brochure by calling 1-800-860-8747.

PUBLICATIONS

Prevent diabetes problems: Keep your feet and skin healthy (2008) [free booklet]. (NIH Publication). National Institutes of Health, accessed November 2007 from http://www.diabetes.niddk.nih.gov/dm/pubs/complications_feet/index.htm, or 1-800-860-8747.

Medicare Coverage of Diabetes Supplies and Services [free booklet]. Centers for Medicare and Medicaid Services (CMS Publication No. 11022): accessed July 2009. http:// www.medicare.gov/health/Diabetes.asp, or 1-800-MEDICARE.

24

What to do when you forget your medications

For a person living with diabetes, you are likely to be keenly aware of the time of day, often asking yourself:

▪ Is it time to test my blood glucose?
▪ Is it time for me to eat?
▪ Is it time for me to take my medication?

Unfortunately, you may not always have the answer. Having a daily plan is the best way to make sure your daily diabetes care tasks are carried out. It doesn't mean that you are now enlisted in a structured boot camp. Instead, it means you have simply thought ahead, so you can decide your strategy for what lies ahead during the day. Ideally, you could have set regular times for:

▪ Testing your blood glucose
▪ Eating
▪ Taking medications

Most diabetes medications should be taken at specific times of day. Medications usually work by helping (in some way) to lower your blood glucose after a meal—therefore, the balance between medication and food is very important. If you eat and do not take your prescribed diabetes medication, you may face a blood glucose level as high as a kite for several hours after a meal. The hyperglycemia may make you feel groggy and cause other symptoms such as a headache or frequent urination.

If you take your prescribed diabetes medications and decide to skip the next meal(s), you may risk having a hypoglycemic event (low blood glucose), depending on the medication. Some medications do not cause hypoglycemia, while others, such as insulin and certain types of diabetes pills, are designed to lower your blood glucose. Without food in your system to balance the medication, your blood glucose could be lowered below normal levels.

Something else to consider: if you're not correctly timing your medication or you're skipping doses, you could be throwing away money! Medications are expensive—if you are going to buy them, get their full value! To do so, make sure you:

✓ Know how they work in your body
✓ Know when to take them
✓ Know how much to take
✓ Know how to get more when you run out

IF YOU FORGET TO TAKE YOUR MEDICATION

Still, no one's perfect. There will be times when you forget or miss a dose. Here are guidelines to help you out:

▮ Know the name of each of your medications (diabetes and others). Unless it is a generic drug, each medication will likely have two names written on the prescription label—a chemical name (what it's made up of) and a marketing name (what the company calls it). If the print is difficult for you to read, ask your pharmacy to print you out a Patient Information Sheet (required by most states) with the information. Asking for help means you have to know what you are asking about.

▮ Learn about medications from a trained health care professional. Most pharmacies offer free patient education with a pharmacist to their customers. If you use more than one pharmacy, consolidate your medication list and share it with each pharmacy to avoid possible drug interactions.

▮ If it has been less than an hour since you were supposed to take your medication, try to call your local pharmacy (24-hour pharmacists may be able to help as well) or health care provider to see if you can take it on a delayed basis. NEVER take a medication on a delayed basis unless you have been instructed by an expert to do so.

■ Check your blood glucose NOW. If it is in a range that you have been instructed to report to your physician, do so. Check your blood glucose several times until your next medication dose is due or your next meal.

■ If it is several hours from when you were to take your medication and you are now ready to take your next usual dose, DO NOT DOUBLE UP on your medication. Always take the recommended dose (not more, not less) unless you have consulted with your medical team.

■ If it is the MIDDLE OF THE NIGHT, and you woke up realizing you forgot, test your blood glucose to see your control. Remember the training you had in diabetes education classes for hyperglycemia (high) and hypoglycemia (low). If you are anxious or have an unusual blood glucose, call your health care provider after-hours support person.

TO AVOID FORGETTING MEDICATIONS

Use reminders to help you stay on track.

■ Set your cell phone to alarm.

■ Many home blood glucose meters and insulin pumps have an "alarm clock" setting—take advantage of this function and use it.

■ Set your computer or cell phone alarm for meal and medication times while you are at work.

■ Set alarm clocks at home.

■ Use pill reminder boxes. Some pharmacies offer a service to pre-fill these in advance, if needed.

■ Use a calendar or diary to mark when you take your medications.

■ Use environmental triggers, such as watching the morning news, to help remind you.

■ Ask a friend or family member to help you stay on track.

Finally, it is not a perfect world. You will forget your medications once in a while—learn to forgive yourself. You can stay prepared by keeping treatments for both hyperglycemia and hypoglycemia on hand at all times, at home and away.

MORE RESOURCES TO EXPLORE

WEBSITES

ForgettingThePill.com . . . . WWW.FORGETTINGTHEPILL.COM
This website offers a number of pill organizers, reminders, and alarms. They also have a toll-free number: 1-877-FORGET2 (367-4382).

e-pill . . . . WWW.EPILL.COM
Another website devoted to pill reminders and organizers. You can also call toll-free 1-800-549-0095.

National Institutes of Health . . . . WWW.DIABETES.NIDDK.NIH.GOV
Website of the NIH and NIDDK, where you can find the free brochure "Medications for People with Diabetes."

National Institutes of Health . . . . WWW.NLM.NIH.GOV
Website of the U.S. National Library and National Institutes of Health, where you can find the brochure "Oral Diabetes Medications," and other publications of the American Academy of Family Physicians.

How to make time for your health

The demands of everyday life create a never-ending task list. If you are a caregiver or parent, not only do you have a list of your needs, but a list of needs of others. Is your health a priority with all the demands you carry each day? Do you make it a priority to perform daily physical activity or make healthy food choices? Despite all the modern conveniences to save time, it seems we have even less of it. When you reflect upon the lifestyles of the early settlers, their main focus was on basic human needs: drawing water from a nearby stream, hunting for food, and maintaining a shelter against nature's elements.

For those of us in the 21st century, if we want water, not only can we simply turn on a faucet, but we frequently use special water filters or bottled spring water to quench our thirst and raise the quality of our water. Food is everywhere in our lives, and you don't even have to cook it; millions of restaurants are available to us if we have a few dollars to spare.

So what have you done with all the time freed up by labor-saving devices and modern conveniences? If providing basic self-care and preventative health measures are not the first things that come to mind, it may be time for you to evaluate your priorities. The number one priority should be taking care of your one and only body, so you can live a long and healthy life. This means taking the time to eat right, exercise, manage your stress, and follow medical and health recommendations.

Parents, spouses and other caregivers often put others' needs in front of their own, and can get lost in the struggle to squeeze 25 hours into a regular day. However, it is not a selfish act to put your own health first, because if you are not well, you can no longer care for others. If you have diabetes, you know there are consequences of not taking care of your body each day, both short-term (feeling tired because your blood glucose is high today) and long-term (chronic complications such as heart disease, kidney disease, eye disease, and other health problems related to poor diabetes control).

QUOTES TO CONSIDER

"The future is here—in the heart of here and now."
—Sri Chinmoy

"No man is rich enough to buy back his past."
—Oscar Wilde

"Nothing is worth more than this day."
—Johann Wolfgang von Goethe

"If you worry about what might be, and wonder what might have been, you will ignore what is."
—Author Unknown

10 SIMPLE STEPS TO HEALTH

Here is a list of 10 preventative steps you can take to have a healthier future.

1. Get moving. Follow a daily physical activity program—period.

2. Quit tobacco. If you smoke, stop—exclamation!

3. Check your A1C to be A-OK. Have an A1C test done regularly and ideally strive to get an A1C of less than 7%, or a level your health care provider promotes. Get an A1C check:

■ At least twice a year if you are meeting your medical treatment goals
■ Quarterly if you are not meeting your medical treatment goals, have had an adjustment in therapy during the year, or have undergone a change in health condition

4. See the future. Have a thorough annual eye exam, including dilation by an optometrist or ophthalmologist. A vision test for eyeglasses is not enough. Your ability to see should be checked and you should receive a full examination to explore the health of your eyes. See your eye specialist as soon as possible if any of the following occur:

- Double vision
- Eye pain
- Eye pressure
- Visible spots, lights, or floaters
- Change in peripheral vision
- Any injury to the eye

5. It might be embarrassing, but it is well worth it. Have your doctor or health care professional check your feet at every visit. At least once a year, they need to perform a comprehensive foot evaluation including:

- Use of a monofilament tool to help assess sensation. This tool is a small handheld device containing a small length of thin plastic of a specific diameter that will be placed on various areas of the foot to determine sensation. Different diameter (thickness) strips may be used to help further evaluate degrees of sensation in an area.
- Tuning fork. A tuning fork can help to diagnose sensory changes in your feet. This non-invasive, painless procedure to evaluate nerve damage uses a small metal two-pronged (not sharp) device shaped like a fork. When the metal fork is tapped against a hard surface, it vibrates. While vibrating, the tuning fork will be placed at different locations on the feet to help determine level of sensation present.
- Palpation of the feet. The clinician will use their hands and possibly small instruments (stethoscope, mirrors, thermometer scans) to inspect the feet and toes. The exam is not limited to examining temperature, assessing pulses, inspecting overall condition of the feet and toes.
- Visual inspection of the entire foot and between toes. Areas with skin breakdown, abnormal growths or calluses, nail deformities, toe deformities, color change, structural changes will be assessed.

6. Stun them with a great smile and fresh breath. Have your teeth cleaned professionally twice a year.

7. Don't let the pressure get to you. Ensure your blood pressure is measured at every visit, with a goal of 130/80 mmHg, as recommended by the American Diabetes Association. Your health care provider may establish different levels for you. Keep track of your levels; if you notice an increase in your numbers, address it with your health care provider.

8. Know your heart attack and stroke risk. People with diabetes are at higher risk for developing heart disease and having a stroke. Exercise, a healthy diet, and regular exams can help prevent these problems from developing. Have a lipid profile performed annually. A lipid profile is a group of blood tests that measure total cholesterol, low-density liproproteins (LDLs, or "bad" cholesterol), high-density liporproteins (HDLs, or "good" cholesterol), and triglycerides (TG).

- ▌Goal for LDL: <100 mg/dl
- ▌Goal for HDL: >40 mg/dl for men
  >50 mg/dl for women
- ▌Goal for TG: <150 mg/dl

9. Pee in a cup. Have a microalbuminuria test (tests protein in the urine) and a glomerular filtration rate (GFR) test. Diabetes can damage how your kidneys work. Kidneys work by filtering waste products out of our blood. High glucose levels over time can damage the filtering process, causing kidney disease to develop. The microalbuminuria and GFR tests can help evaluate your kidney function and determine the presence of kidney disease. Kidney disease can progress to a point where the kidneys stop working properly. If this happens, a kidney transplant or artificial kidney systems (dialysis) will be required to sustain life. Diabetes is the leading cause of new kidney disease cases in the United States. The best way to help prevent kidney disease from starting is to keep your blood glucose and blood pressure in the "good" range established by your health care professionals.

10. Be proactive. Discuss the need for other preventative measures with your physician, such as:

- Aspirin therapy
- Preventative blood pressure medications
- Preventative cholesterol medications
- Annual flu shot
- Annual pneumonia shot
- Birth control and pre-pregnancy planning
- Weight maintenance tips and strategies

MORE RESOURCES TO EXPLORE

WEBSITES

National Diabetes Education Program. . . . . . WWW.NDEP.NIH.GOV
Website for the National Diabetes Education Program, where you can find the free brochure "4 Steps to Control Your Diabetes." You can also have a copy sent to you by calling 1-800-438-5383.

American Diabetes Association . . . . WWW.DIABETES.ORG
Website of the American Diabetes Association, which includes information on Make the Link! Diabetes, Heart Disease and Stroke. You can get more information by calling 1-800-DIABETES.

Diabetes PhD . . . . WWW.DIABETES.ORG/PHD
Website for Diabetes PhD, an interactive health-monitoring program for people with diabetes. It can help you track your annual exam information and provide insight into risks of chronic complications.

BOOKS

The Uncomplicated Guide to Diabetes Complications, 3rd edition, by Marvin E. Levin and Michael A. Pfeifer. American Diabetes Association; Alexandria, VA, 2009.

CHAPTER 6

WHAT ELSE CAN AFFECT YOUR BLOOD GLUCOSE?

26
How tobacco affects diabetes

Tobacco products, whether smokeless or not, will negatively affect your overall health, including your diabetes care. Using tobacco products causes your blood glucose to increase, obstructing your efforts to control your diabetes. In addition, using tobacco problems will cause you to have a greater chance of developing diabetes complications, heart disease, or lung disease or having a stroke as well as certain forms of cancer. The average smoker has probably contemplated giving up cigarettes several times, but may not have had enough motivation and/or support to be successful.

THE FEAR FACTOR

Thinking about quitting smoking can actually cause anxious feelings in some individuals. How will I do it? How will I cope if I can't smoke? What if I gain a lot of weight? What if I fail? These emotional concerns are important and need to be addressed with your health care professional honestly. There is a myth that only "some people" have the ability to quit and others don't. You can do it, but it will require making a commitment, creating and implementing a plan, and obtaining support from your family, friends, and health care team.

Your family and health care team may be dealing with some of their own fears. They have fears for your future health. Hopefully, their feelings and concerns about smoking will be shared with you respectfully, rather than in a threatening manner. But, let's face it: the threat of smoking to your health is very serious.

- **Save your feet:** Tobacco use impairs the circulation in smaller blood vessels, which are present in the feet and legs. Having circulation problems in your feet and legs will increase your risk of foot ulcers, lower-extremity infections, and amputations.
- **Save your kidneys:** Tobacco use causes an increase in blood pressure, which creates an added strain on your kidneys. Some resources state smoking triples the risk of developing diabetes kidney disease (nephropathy). The kidneys' role in the body is to filter fluids so that wastes are removed and eliminated. If this function is impaired, kidney disease will result and may lead to complete kidney failure. Artificial dialysis will be needed for survival when kidney disease progresses.
- **Save your eyes:** Smoking can increase problems with retinopathy (an eye disease affecting the retina) as well as macular degeneration.
- **Save your heart:** Research indicates you are about three times more likely to die of heart disease if you have diabetes and you use tobacco products.
- **Save your teeth and breath:** Smoking or chewing tobacco will affect your oral health and further increase your risk of gum disease and damage to teeth. Smoking not only makes your breath stink, it causes you to have a harder time breathing upon exertion, since it affects your lung function.
- **Save your nervous system:** Smoking will increase the risk of having neuropathy (damage to your nerves), which can affect how your body parts feel, how your stomach empties, how your body's sexual organs function, and how your bladder and bowel function.
- **Save your life:** Smoking reduces your life expectancy.

ARE YOU READY TO QUIT?

This is the key question you should ask yourself before attempting this lifestyle change. If you are not, perhaps in the near future you will be. Become more educated on the effects of tobacco on your health and about local resources while you are waiting for the best time. Choose a time to make this lifestyle change when you are not already dealing with other life stressors or major changes. If you are ready, start building a support team. First, discuss your idea with your family and friends. Get them on board. Next, consult a health care professional about the various methods to help you with tobacco cessation:

■ Nicotine replacement therapy (patches, gums, lozenges, inhalers, sprays)
■ Smoking cessation programs
■ Counseling
■ Medications

WHAT SHOULD I EXPECT FROM A QUALITY SMOKING CESSATION PROGRAM?

■ Education on benefits of smoking cessation
■ A leader who has specialized training in smoking cessation
■ Support/reward system
■ Strategies to deal with withdrawal symptoms (physical and psychological)
■ Relapse prevention strategies
■ No selling or pushing you to buy expensive tools, food, or supplemental products
■ A follow-up process
■ Information and strategies to minimize risk of subsequent weight gain and depression

WHAT ABOUT SMOKELESS TOBACCO PRODUCTS?

If you chew or dip tobacco, you will likely experience higher blood glucose levels, not just from the tobacco, but from the flavoring agents used in making the product. In addition, the tobacco can greatly increase your risk of gum, teeth, and mouth problems.

WHAT ARE THE REWARDS?

■ On the first day, heart rate improves, blood pressure drops, carbon monoxide levels drop, and circulation improves.
■ Breath/clothes/hair/skin smell better.
■ After 1 year, the extra risk of heart disease drops to 50% of what it was when you were a smoker.
■ Risk of lung cancer decreases.
■ Risk of circulatory and diabetes complication disorders decrease.

- Lung function improves.
- Looks improve (smoking causes stinky hair, yellowed skin/fingernails).
- You have extra money.
- Life expectancy improves—now that's value!

MORE RESOURCES TO EXPLORE

WHERE CAN I FIND RESOURCES?

Check with your health care professional about local programs. Many local health departments, extension services, and local hospitals provide smoking cessation classes. If you have computer access, try these resources:

WEBSITES

American Diabetes Association . . . . WWW.DIABETES.ORG/
TYPE-1-DIABETES/SMOKING.JSP
This section of the American Diabetes Association website gives a good overview of how smoking adversely affects your diabetes management, and gives information on how to quit.

American Heart Association . . . . WWW.AMHRT.ORG
Website of the American Heart Association.

Centers for Disease Control . . . . WWW.CDC.GOV/TOBACCO
This section of the Centers for Disease Control and Prevention website is devoted to Smoking and Health.

American Lung Association . . . . WWW.LUNGUSA.ORG
Freedom From Smoking (online program), an initiative of the American Lung Association.

National Cancer Institute . . . . WWW.CANCER.GOV
Website for the National Cancer Institute.

NO COMPUTER? TRY TELEPHONE HELP LINES

Tobacco Quit Line, 1-888-567-TRUTH,
Tobacco Prevention and Control Program

Quitline, American Cancer Society, 1-800-ACS-2345

Nicotine Anonymous, 1-877-879-6422

Smoking Cessation Leadership Center, 1-800-QUITNOW

How your menstrual cycle affects your blood glucose

The natural changes in female hormones, which control a woman's monthly cycle, have an impact on another hormone—insulin. It seems diabetes seems to get in the way of just about everything. Instead of tossing your hands up in the air, thinking you are helpless to battle with another one of your hormones acting up, learn how you can face the challenge and conquer.

The primary female hormone is estrogen, which actually represents a group of steroid compounds produced by the ovaries. Another hormone produced by the ovaries is progesterone. During each monthly cycle, the amount of these hormones (estrogen and progesterone) present in the blood changes. When the level of these hormones changes, particularly in the second half of each woman's monthly cycle, many women report seeing a trend in their blood glucose logs, and not a positive one. Theories suggest the rise and fall of the hormones of estrogen and progesterone create a problem of more insulin resistance in the body, resulting in higher blood glucose levels at certain times of the month. Some women experience high blood glucose levels just before their period and then experience hypoglycemia during their period.

Therefore, every woman's cycle is unique, and it cannot be predicted that every woman will experience hyperglycemia only at one phase of the monthly cycle. Instead, if you think your blood glucose may be affected, try the following strategies (see box).

If PMS or your cycle is hindering your normal lifestyle demands, or is creating significant problems with your blood

GATHER INFORMATION TO TEST YOUR THEORY OVER A FEW MONTHS:

▮ Check your blood glucose frequently 3–5 days before the onset of your cycle.

▮ Check your blood glucose frequently the day of the onset of your period.

▮ Check your blood glucose regularly through your period.

▮ Check your blood glucose frequently a few days after your period stops.

▮ TIP: In doing this, try to be consistent with your documentation, noting whether the test result is a fasting result, or before or after a meal, so that your information can be compared to identify trends.

Compare your blood glucose logs to each other, noting your monthly cycle to see if you can see a pattern that has developed. Share this information with your health care provider.

IF YOU SUFFER FROM PMS SYMPTOMS (FATIGUE, CRAMPING, BLOATING, HEADACHES, ETC.)

Try some of these strategies to reduce your symptoms:

▮ Stick with your meal plan.

▮ Engage in regular physical activity.

▮ See if cutting back on certain types of foods helps improve symptoms (avoiding alcohol, too much caffeine, and sodium may help).

▮ Practice stress management.

Create a plan for dealing with those high blood glucose days:

▮ Discuss changes to your long-acting or short-acting insulin regime (if applicable) with your health care provider for the days you anticipate higher-than-normal readings. Create a flexible plan, since you may experience different degrees of elevations month by month.

▮ If you wear a pump, learn how to use temporary basal rates to adjust your basal settings for short periods of time, or several days.

▮ Watch out for food cravings. Make sure you stocked the pantry with low-calorie or low-carbohydrate snack choices so that you can fix the problem of the munchies without causing even more hyperglycemia problems.

- Stay physically active.

- Stay hydrated.

- Try to stay on your normal meal plan. Having PMS symptoms may increase or decrease your appetite. This can create further swings in your blood glucose. You may find benefits in your symptoms by choosing whole-grain and higher-fiber products and less refined foods.

- Achieve pain control. Pain can also contribute to high blood glucose levels. If you suffer from cramping, ask your physician what pain medications you should be using to help manage your pain.

- Discuss with your registered dietitian if it may be beneficial to adjust your meal plan (or carbohydrate-to-insulin ratios if used) to avoid high or low blood glucose problems during your cycle.

- Keep plenty of extra strips on hand for those days you may be increasing your testing frequency.

glucose control, seek a medical evaluation from a gynecologist to help investigate the source of the continuing problem. For example, polycystic ovarian syndrome (PCOS) is a common problem where ovulation is impaired. This syndrome has been clearly associated with insulin resistance and has been treated successfully through various treatment options. PCOS is often improved with weight loss, regular physical activity, and a healthy meal plan. Some individuals may take oral diabetes medications, which have been shown to reduce symptoms and improve insulin sensitivity.

TIP: All women with diabetes within childbearing age should discuss options for either planning or preventing pregnancy with their health care provider at least annually.

MORE RESOURCES TO EXPLORE

BOOKS

Sex and Diabetes, by Janis Roszler and Donna Rice. American Diabetes Association; Alexandria, VA, 2007.

Sex and Diabetes. This chapter can be found in *The Complete Guide to Diabetes,* 4th edition. American Diabetes Association; Alexandria, VA, 2005.

Women and Diabetes: Life Planning for Health and Wellness, by Linda M. Poirier. American Diabetes Association; Alexandria, VA, 1997.

WEBSITES

Polycystic Ovarian Syndrome
  Association . . . . WWW.PCOSUPPORT.ORG.
  Website of the Polycystic Ovarian Syndrome Association.

DiabetesNet . . . . WWW.DIABETESNET.COM/DIABETES_INFORMATION/
                                    DIABETES_WOMEN.PHP
  This link takes you to Women and Diabetes, The Menstrual Cycle and Diabetes, a section of the DiabetesNet website.

How to do ketone testing

Ketones are just one more thing to keep up with. Ketone bodies (acetone, aceto-acetic acid, and beta-hydroxybutyric acid) are waste products resulting from times when the body uses fat instead of glucose as an alternative fuel source. When your metabolism is working normally, available glucose nourishes the body. For the body to use the glucose, insulin must be present and working properly.

In diabetes, insulin is either no longer being made (as in type 1) or it is not working as well as it should for various reasons (as in type 2 and gestational diabetes). The body has a never-ending need for fuel. If glucose is not readily available, a cry for nourishment by the cells results in the body tapping into reserved energy sources in the body—fat cells.

Ketones are a waste product resulting from the use of fat within the body. Fat cells can be converted into glucose; however, this metabolic process produces a harmful byproduct—ketones. This is the tradeoff for getting fuel. Think about gasoline-powered vehicles—we need gasoline to get them to go, but then we get a toxic waste product (exhaust fumes) that we have to get rid of in the process.

In the human body, if ketones were left to build up in the body, serious consequences would result. The condition associated with the buildup of ketones in the blood is known as diabetic ketoacidosis, or DKA. Some individuals refer to this as "diabetic coma," a life-threatening condition.

As a rule, small amounts of body fat are used without any problem in humans, such as when a person with normal metabolism skips a meal, or delays eating, or has a sudden demand for a great deal of energy. The body in this example is not at risk of having problems with ketones, because it was a limited amount of time, and the individual had a healthy metabolism to make sure balance is restored. Ketones are normally quickly excreted through the urine, to dispose of this waste product.

Unfortunately, in diabetes, when your body burns too much fat because of energy imbalances, or there is not enough insulin to meet the body's basic needs, ketones may be produced in a large enough amount that the levels build up in the bloodstream. The body simply cannot get rid of the ketones fast enough through the urine.

Because ketone bodies start to appear in the urine, home test kits were developed decades ago to help individuals test themselves for the presence of ketones. Your insurance company may or may not cover the cost of these strips; call to find out if a prescription is needed for coverage or if it will be out of pocket. Regardless of the cost, individuals with type 1 diabetes and pregnant women with diabetes (type 1, type 2, and gestational diabetes) should have test strips as a standard diabetes supply item in the home.

Urine ketone test kits are simply small plastic dipsticks with a small test pad area on one end. The test pad contains chemical agents within the pad, and in an unused state, has a neutral color appearance. If ketones are present, once exposed to a sample, the test pad will change color. To do the test, the individual needs to take out a test strip. The test pad is saturated with urine (either by dipping it into a sample contained in a clean cup or passing it through the urine stream). After waiting the appropriate amount of time as specified on the manufacturer's directions, the color of the test pad is compared to a color chart. The color correlates to a specific level of ketones, as indicated by a result scale usually printed on the vial of strips, or within the package instructions. The results are often reported by descriptive terms such as "trace," "small," "moderate," or "large," but also may be accompanied by laboratory values (numbers) such as 5, 15, 50, or 80 mg/dl.

IS URINE TESTING ACCURATE?

With any home testing products, there is the possibility of errors in testing. For urine ketone testing, some of the following situations may result in inaccurate results:

- Outdated strips used (always check the manufacturer's dates before use)
- Opened strips will expire after a certain amount of time. Read the label to determine the shelf life of the strips once opened. TIP: Some ketone strips are packaged individually in foil wrappers—using these strips can save you money if you test for ketones infrequently.
- Improper storage of strips (too hot or cold). Follow storage guidelines; if the strips have been exposed to moisture, heat, or cold, the integrity of the strips will be affected.
- Do not touch the test pad area or lay it on a surface before testing, since it could become reactive to the environmental influence and impair testing.
- Some prescribed medications may affect test strips (check with your pharmacist).
- Hydration may affect results (dehydration may cause a false-positive result).
- Individuals who are color-blind (those who cannot discern colors) should have someone else interpret results.
- Urine is produced and stored in the bladder. If the individual has not emptied the bladder for a prolonged period of time, the results are not likely indicative of the current status.

IS THERE ANOTHER WAY TO TEST FOR KETONES?

At present, there is one blood glucose meter that can be used to test for blood ketones as well as blood glucose. The product is called Precision Xtra and is currently made by Abbott Diagnostics. Check with your doctor if he or she prefers urine testing or blood testing for ketones. Having two types of meters may be problematic, since both supplies may not be covered by your insurance, or at the same rate.

WHO SHOULD TEST FOR KETONES?

- Individuals with type 1 diabetes should test when their blood glucose is high, usually >240 mg/dl.
- If you have type 1 diabetes, ask your health care professional

when he or she expects you to perform testing. All people with diabetes who are sick, or who have repeated high blood glucose levels, should test for ketones. Illness causes a greater stress on the body and a greater need for energy—if you are not eating normally, the chance of having a fuel imbalance increases. You may be at risk for both hypoglycemia (low blood glucose complication) as well as ketosis (high blood glucose complication).

▮ Women with diabetes who are pregnant, either with type 1, type 2, or gestational diabetes, should test for urine ketones according to health care professional recommendations.

▮ Sometimes individuals with type 2 diabetes need to test for ketones. Ask your health care provider if you need to.

WHAT ARE THE SYMPTOMS OF DKA?

✓ Unusually high blood glucose readings
✓ Nausea
✓ Vomiting
✓ Feeling lethargic/flu-like feeling
✓ Unusual breathing (fast, shallow)
✓ Extreme thirst
✓ Frequent urination
✓ Headache or abdominal pain

WHAT SHOULD YOU DO IF YOU HAVE KETONES?

If you have ketones, notify your health care provider and follow your health care professional's guidelines. Having ketones is a stressful event for the individual as well as the caregivers. Ideally, ketone testing and interventions for results should be discussed with you at a routine office appointment or through a diabetes education class or session. Knowing what to do at home will give you the opportunity to start treatment immediately to speed your recovery. If DKA is not treated effectively or quickly, it can become a life-threatening situation. If an individual is not able to provide self-care and suspects he or she has DKA, or the individual has not been successful with interventions to improve the situation, outside emergency help should be contacted immediately.

CAN I PREVENT DKA?

Yes, you have the ability to prevent DKA by keeping your blood glucose levels in an acceptable range through your daily management activities. By becoming knowledgeable about what to do in case of severe or persistent hyperglycemia (the root cause of DKA) in advance with your health care provider, you will be able to take action if you detect ketones.

Ketones may result during the following situations:

✓ Frequent high blood glucose levels >240 mg/dl
✓ Illness
✓ Pregnancy
✓ Inadequate medication to control blood glucose levels
✓ Skipping insulin injections
✓ Not taking enough insulin
✓ Not enough basal insulin (such as N, Lantus, or Levemir) to fuel the body
✓ Blocked or dislocated insulin pump catheter (prevents insulin flow)
✓ Expired insulin used
✓ Extreme physical or mental stress events
✓ Damaged strips providing false normal results, when blood glucose is actually very high
✓ Sudden growth
✓ Drug interaction with your diabetes medications, preventing them from working
✓ Ignoring persistent high blood glucose problems
✓ Dehydration

WHAT CAN I DO IF I HAVE A POSITIVE URINE KETONE TEST?

Even at a trace amount level, your health care team will generally recommend the following:

■ Resolving the hyperglycemia immediately with additional insulin (the amount to be determined by your health care professional)
■ Pushing large amounts of water and other non-caloric beverages to help flush the ketones from your system

- Monitoring blood glucose and urine ketones frequently for several hours or longer, to make sure the ketones are history
- Calling to report your progress and situation periodically

MORE RESOURCES TO EXPLORE

MAGAZINES, JOURNALS, AND OTHER PERIODICALS

Urine Testing Products for Ketones and Glucose. 2007 Resource Guide, *Diabetes Forecast*, January 2007. American Diabetes Association; Alexandria, VA.

BOOK

The Complete Guide to Diabetes. 4th edition. American Diabetes Association; Alexandria, VA, 2005.

WEBSITES

American Diabetes Association . . . . WWW.DIABETES.ORG
Website of the American Diabetes Association.

Bayer . . . . WWW.BAYERDIABETES.COM/US
Website of Bayer.

Abbott . . . . WWW.ABBOTTDIABETESCARE.COM
Website of Abbott, maker of the Precision Xtra.

29
How to take the fear out of hypoglycemia

If you talk to others with diabetes, you will often hear about their trials with blood glucose control. Often, the story will begin with, "One time, I even got down as low as...." For many people, hypoglycemia is something to be feared. There are also misconceptions about hypoglycemia, since some still refer to a severe low blood glucose reaction as "diabetic coma." Diabetic coma is in fact a nickname given to the syndrome of extremely high blood glucose compounded by lack of insulin, known as diabetic ketoacidosis (DKA).

Part of the reason individuals fear hypoglycemia is from hearing stories from friends and family members who may have heard the stories of "my worst low." Another reason is likely due to physiology—a person is usually more likely to feel symptoms (weak, shaky, sweaty, lightheaded, nausea, or other) when the blood glucose level drops below normal levels, versus when the blood glucose is climbing. These symptoms may come on slowly or suddenly and create a feeling of anxiousness and discomfort in most people. Individuals will want to resolve the symptoms right away, especially if out in public, because of the social implications of the situation.

It seems strange that if your blood glucose is 20 points lower than normal (say, 50 mg/dl), you can feel really rotten. But you can blaze right on when your blood glucose is 20 points higher than normal (say, about 160 mg/dl). The human body tends to sound an alarm when blood glucose levels are low, so the owner of the body will seek out help to recover from the lack of fuel. Symptoms of even mild hypoglycemia (blood glucose is <70 mg/dl and you are having symptoms, but you are still alert, oriented, and can swallow on your own) are usually quite unpleasant, and many people react to the situation with a sense of panic. The panic can sometimes be acted out in various ways, such as:

- Unnecessary trips to the local emergency room (you may drop lower waiting your turn to be seen, when a home treatment would suffice)
- Unnecessary 911 calls
- Overtreatment of hypoglycemia (three glasses of juice with sugar added)
- Incorrect treatment of hypoglycemia (eating everything and anything in sight, which will perhaps cause a delayed treatment followed later by a huge rise in blood glucose)
- Anger or inappropriate behavior toward the person who is trying to help you

While it is true you should treat hypoglycemia as quickly as possible, there are some prevention steps as well as preparation steps you can do to take the fear out of hypoglycemia.

PREVENTING AND PREPARING FOR HYPOGLYCEMIA

10 TIPS FOR PREVENTION

1. **Check.** Check your blood glucose regularly to catch problems before they happen.

2. **Be on time for dinner.** Don't skip scheduled meals or snacks.

3. **Medicines are meant to alter your body.** Take medications as directed, on time, and the correct amount.

4. **Root canal days.** Consume alternative calorie-containing liquids on days you cannot consume your usual solid foods (such as a sick day, dental treatment day, etc.).

5. **Beep, beep, beep.** Watch your clock during the day to help you stick to your diabetes care routine. Program your watch, clock, cell phone, insulin pump, or computer to send you reminders to stay on track.

6. **Time to go to school.** Learn about diabetes care in a diabetes class from a qualified diabetes educator or health care professional, rather than your neighbor or coworker.

7. **Following your dining experience, walk.** Time your exercise routine to start after a meal, rather than before, so that you have fuel in your system to balance the burning of the fuel when you exercise. This is a new way to look at the phrase "feel the burn!" when you exercise.

8. **Superhuman ego.** Don't overdo physical activities. Physical activities help lower your blood glucose, but don't go on with a new routine or a household chore if you are not sure how it will affect your blood glucose during the activity and after. Don't be superhuman and try to rake "just a few more bags" if you have already been hard at it and it is growing close to mealtime—a time when your energy levels are naturally going to be lower. Physical activity will help lower your blood glucose for several hours after as well, so take along the meter and test *before, during*, and *after* just to see how your blood glucose responds.

9. **Unravel a mystery.** Write down information about the situation when you do have hypoglycemia so that you can play detective later to determine what happened. You might not have been aware of circumstances at the time, but later when you are feeling better, you may be able to help identify causes, which will help you develop a prevention plan.

10. **The tips of my ears get hot.** Know your symptoms—pay attention to how you feel when your blood glucose starts to go down to below normal levels. When you feel them the next time, you will know to check your blood glucose to see what is really going on. Sometimes feeling tired is just because you are tired,

not because you are hypoglycemic. Symptoms are good indicators and vary from person to person, but testing is the most accurate method to determine your glucose level.

10 TIPS FOR PREPARATION

1. **"Honey, don't forget to take your sugar."** Always carry hypoglycemia treatments with you when you leave home. Good choices are:
   ■ Glucose tablets
   ■ Glucose gels
   ■ Juice boxes
   ■ Cake decorating gels
   ■ Regular sodas
   ■ Honey packets from restaurants

   A follow-up snack may or may not be needed. Most health care providers advise you to eat a snack after treating hypoglycemia if you:
   ■ are exercising
   ■ performing a sport
   ■ doing strenuous physical activity
   ■ unable to plan/determine when your next meal will be
   ■ driving
   ■ prone to having moderate to severe hypoglycemia

2. **Restrict the midnight kitchen raiders.** Keep hypoglycemia treatments in the home. Make sure they are "safe" from midnight snackers in the household or insatiable kids. You may want to put your treatment items in a plain paper bag or resealable plastic bag and label it "HYPOGLYCEMIA KIT—DO NOT EAT."

3. **What was this animal?** Check your hypoglycemia treatment kits often to make sure you don't have expired or undesirable food stuffs (crushed, crumbled, otherwise mangled animal crackers, graham crackers, pretzels, etc.) after time passes.

4. **Treat emergencies at home only if you can.** Talk to your doctor about your possible need to have a glucagon emergency kit in the home. Have a family member or friend learn how to use it safely, as well as *when* to use it.

5. **Three stages of the "lows."** Educate yourself on how to treat the three types of hypoglycemia from a trained diabetes educator or health care professional. There is:
   - *Mild* hypoglycemia (conscious, alert, oriented, can swallow)
   - *Moderate* hypoglycemia (conscious but disoriented, may resist attempts to treat from others, can be confused or combative)
   - *Severe* hypoglycemia (unconscious)

6. **Be a teacher.** Train friends, family members, neighbors, roommates, teachers, soccer coaches, ballet teachers, piano teachers, babysitters, and anyone else involved in direct care of the person with diabetes on how to take care of a hypoglycemia reaction.

7. **Pitch your old girlfriend's number and add in 911.** Keep emergency phone numbers on speed dial on landlines and cell phones.

8. **Minutes that seem like eternity.** Recognize there will be a time interval to feeling better after ingestion of a hypoglycemia treatment. It should take only 5–10 minutes, but this seems like eternity to some. Chugging 64 ounces of juice is not a good idea if you don't feel instantly better. Resist the temptation to over-treat. Wait 5–10 minutes and treat your other symptoms, such as putting a cool cloth on your head, sitting down, loosening clothing, or whatever makes you feel comfortable. Portion your treatment items in advance, if possible, such as prepared juice boxes, sports drinks, or lunchbox-size soda cans, all about 4–6 ounces in size.

9. **Save the boxing gloves.** Know that you may have to have others help you if your hypoglycemia is more than mild. Talk about your preferred treatments, so that there is no conflict over what type of juice, or how cold it is, or how much you will need during a hypoglycemic event. An argument will just make the situation worse.

10. **Feeling worried.** Talk to your health care professional if you have anxious feelings or serious worries about hypoglycemia. Ignore the stories from the beauty shop or auto parts shop—those are not the best places to get medical advice!

MORE RESOURCES TO EXPLORE

WEBSITES

Children with Diabetes . . . . WWW.CHILDRENWITHDIABETES.COM
  Especially helpful is the "Hypoglycemia" section of this website.

National Diabetes Information

Clearinghouse . . . . HTTP://DIABETES.NIDDK.NIH.GOV/
DM/PUBS/HYPOGLYCEMIA/
  This link will take you to the "Hypoglycemia" section of the National Diabetes Information Clearinghouse website, a division of the NIH.

PRODUCTS

Glucagon Emergency Kit, manufactured by Eli Lilly and Company.

GlucaGen HypoKit, manufactured by Novo Nordisk Pharmaceuticals.

30

What to do about roller coaster readings

Your body is unique—there is not another one like it anywhere in the world. How your blood glucose responds to certain types of food, activity, stress, and illness will also be unique. This means you need to work closely with your health care provider so your care can be individualized. Don't expect your doctor to give you the perfect plan right off the bat. That's like expecting you to be "perfect" right off with your management as well. It is also not enough to go for a yearly checkup and expect your health care provider to "straighten out" your blood glucose levels that have been going haywire for months. Most health care providers ask their patients with diabetes to come for quarterly visits, but if your blood glucose levels are not within target, or you are having treatment adjustments, they may ask for you to come monthly.

Information from your food diaries, blood glucose records, and personal calendar (tracking special days, work shift changes, menstrual cycle dates, etc.) will all help you uncover facts to determine the source of roller coaster

HOW TO HELP STRAIGHTEN OUT ROLLER COASTER READINGS

DO:

✓ Test your blood glucose as directed (two to four times a day is usually expected).

✓ When visiting your health care professional, take in your blood glucose diary or meter, which can be downloaded.

✓ Make notes in your diary of special situations, as well as mark whether the readings were before meals or after (obviously, before-meal readings should be a bit lower, and there are expected goal ranges for both situations).

✓ Discuss any concerns you have.

✓ Share information about any trends you may have discovered on your own.

✓ Reveal any unexpected events that occurred such as vacation time, sick time, etc.

✓ Carry a positive attitude and be willing to try new treatment strategies.

✓ Take someone with you if you tend to forget the recommendations, or write them down during your visit.

DON'T:

✓ Go to the appointment without any written data, or with fragments of data or food diaries, and throw your hands in the air and say, "I can't do anything about my blood glucose levels, and you need to fix it." It takes a team and real information to make improvements.

blood glucose readings. The box above contains some examples of how information can help smooth out the twists, turns, climbs, and dives of diabetes control.

TWO EXAMPLES OF HOW GOOD INFORMATION GATHERING CAN HELP

MIKE

His statement: "I don't know why my blood glucose is fine one morning, and the next morning it is high. It is just out of control."

His diabetes plan: 20 units of Lantus at bedtime, 1,000 mg metformin every morning

His blood glucose log:

Sun	Mon	Tues	Wed	Thurs	Fri	Sat
925 am: 135 took pills	709 am: 205 took pills	711 am: 129 took pills	715 am: 119 took pills	705 am: 160 took pills	655 am: 98 took pills	930 am: 77 took pills
501 pm: 169	530 pm: 188	5 pm: 135	6 pm: 127	530 pm: 133	545 pm: 125	7 pm: 98
1115 pm: 215 injected Lantus	903 pm: 143 injected Lantus	830 pm: 150 injected Lantus	1006 pm: 203 injected Lantus	9 pm: 139 injected Lantus	1130 pm: 285 injected Lantus	1145 pm: 140 injected Lantus

Rewind

1st observation: Lantus is being taken at different times. Lantus is a long-acting insulin and has an ~24-hour effect. By taking it at various times (as much as 3 or more hours difference if you read the log), there may be times you will have gaps or overlap in coverage, which can result in rises and falls.

2nd observation: Mike's weekday schedule is different from his weekend schedule. He needs to discuss the differences in his waking/sleeping schedule as well as food behaviors (meal and snack choices and times) on these different days. It is doubtful his doctor will force him to conform to one schedule 24/7. Rather, he or she will work with Mike to customize the right plan for better consistency.

3rd observation: Food intake is not recorded, so it is difficult to see what effect food choices and timing have on his readings. Mike's health care provider will likely ask for food records the next time.

4th observation: Mike takes insulin by injection. Swings in blood glucose level can be caused by inaccurate insulin measuring technique, changing the injection site, or improper injection technique. Sometimes you can be going so fast to get the injection done, you may not realize you made an error. The type of syringe can make a difference as well (for comfort, there are some fine needle syringes out there), but if you have tough skin, or are overusing the same injection site, the insulin may not be in the adipose tissue area (fatty tissue) just under the skin. Make sure you rotate your sites. Right-handed people tend to abuse the "left side" of their abdomen, whereas the lefties do the opposite. Finally, in some cases, insulin is injected by insulin injection devices. There are proper procedures for using insulin-pen delivery devices that differ from syringe injections; make sure you know each step.

5th observation: The big unknown: what is happening during the sleeping hours? It may be a good idea for Mike to test eight times a day for a few days to get some more numbers. For instance, checking before each meal, 2 hours after each meal, at bedtime, and between 2:00 and 3:00 a.m. will help give more information.

DEBRA

Her statement: "I can eat the same thing, and my blood glucose is always different."

Her diabetes plan: No medications.

Her blood glucose results: Didn't bring them.

Rewind

1st observation: Many people enjoy the same favorite sandwich for lunch or same favorite cereal for breakfast. However, what they don't always take into account are the following possible factors:

- Quantity—Unless you measure each and every time, your quantities can be different.
- Combinations—Small changes such as having a small apple versus a large banana, even though they are both fruits, may have an effect on your blood glucose. The carbohydrate content and quantity can affect your postmeal readings. Higher fat will cause a higher postmeal reading, but not until several hours later, so a choice of having baked chips or regular chips can also affect your readings.
- Activity—Your activity causes your blood glucose levels to change, and each day you certainly have different activity. Even parking in a close spot to work one day and a farther one another day can have an effect on your blood glucose, or doing laundry one day after dinner and relaxing in a chair

instead the next. Exercise sometimes can affect a person's blood glucose several hours later. Keeping details on your day will help provide clues to your rises and falls.

■ Physical condition—Your body chemistry will also have an influence. Changes such as illness, menstrual cycle, pain (such as migraines), and other factors can affect your blood glucose.

■ Alcohol—If you consume alcohol, it can affect your blood glucose several hours later by lowering it. This is caused by the alcohol interfering with your metabolism (the way you use your food energy).

■ Stress—Your body responds to physical and mental stress by altering your blood glucose. Dealing with bad news or a difficult challenge at school or work can be enough to cause some internal stress, which can silently cause a high blood glucose reaction.

■ Blood glucose checks—Are your blood glucose checks being done at the same time? Ideally, to see how a meal affects your blood glucose, you should check before the meal (and before taking your premeal medication, if prescribed). Then wait 2 hours after to recheck. Timing is everything. If you check only 90 minutes after a meal one day, and 3 hours after a meal another, you are comparing apples to oranges.

■ Premeal blood glucose level—Was your premeal blood glucose the same *before* the meal? If your blood glucose was more than 10–15% different going *in* to the meal, even if you consume the same microwaveable low-calorie dinner plate, your blood glucose will be different going *out* of the meal.

■ Strips and your technique—Testing with expired strips, or not getting enough blood, can also affect your readings.

> **TIP:** Find someone who is willing to spend the time looking at your home data, listen to your reports, and ask you questions, rather than just reading your A1C level.

2nd observation: Can't complete a good evaluation without the data—bring your blood glucose records and food diaries to your visits if you want more than speculation.

MORE RESOURCES TO EXPLORE

BOOKS

101 Tips for Improving Blood Glucose, 2nd edition, by David Schade. American Diabetes Association; Alexandria, VA, 1999.

Fast Facts: Playing the Numbers, by Laurinda Poirier-Solomon. American Diabetes Association; Alexandria, VA, 2003.

The Complete Guide to Diabetes, 4th edition. American Diabetes Association; Alexandria, VA, 2007.

CHAPTER 7

DEAL WITH SPECIAL HEALTH ISSUES

31

How to prevent recurring infections

Having an imbalance of your blood glucose will also create an imbalance in your body's ability to heal minor injuries and fight off nasty infections. There are two main reasons for this problem: 1) the body's natural immune system (defense system) is impaired when glucose levels are high, and 2) germs, fungal bodies, and other "cooties" love sugar, too, and will grow quickly if blood glucose levels are high (more food equals better growth). While it is true that germs are everywhere, and you even have some living on your body and in your home all the time, it is important to try to prevent an infection from getting started. Infections can be difficult to treat, even with today's antibiotics and drugs. This is even truer when you have diabetes.

Let's think about how our body reacts to a germ-fighting need, such as responding to a cut on your big toe, where outside germs could easily enter. Inside our body, our bloodstream is like small highways or hallways. There are all sorts of travelers in these byways, such as red blood cells (which carry oxygen), vitamins and minerals (to keep us strong), fluids (to move things along and keep us hydrated), glucose (blood glucose/fuel for the body), and white blood cells (which help fight off infections). White blood cells are big and like to move smoothly along.

Let's look at an example of how our bloodstream works, with an example of how the traffic flow works. Think about what it is like when the lunch bell rings in a typical junior high school—the halls immediately get filled with kids, all trying to get to the same spot. Somehow, they all manage to get there, with some likely shoving and pushing each and every day. And everyone gets their fill of fish fingers and French fries.

Imagine now on another day that you add more travelers in the system (such as when you have hyperglycemia, you are adding more glucose into the bloodstream). Suddenly, a warning comes across the loudspeaker for everyone to run to the cafeteria. The speaker implores all the school inhabitants to hurry up, since the cafeteria is running an emergency special on ice cream. The freezer broke and the ice cream will melt quickly, causing a gooey mess that may cause damage in the main kitchen. Suddenly, the halls are jam-packed with lots of these extra glucose bodies running around. The larger white blood cell travelers are in a bind—they cannot move well because of the crowd, and they don't perform well navigating around all the chaos. These larger cells can eat more than the rest and would be a great help to resolve the problem quickly. But, by the time they get to the cafeteria, the crisis of melted rocky road ice cream may be a reality if they can't get there and do their part. Or, if they get bumped and bruised up along the way and feel too weakened to help once they get there.

Okay, so that was a bit of a stretch, but hopefully, you can understand a little more why people with diabetes have a higher risk of infection. The key points to reduce risk of infections are as follows:

1. Practice good body hygiene.
2. Maintain a healthy immune system.
3. Maintain good blood glucose control.
4. Treat minor problems quickly and correctly.
5. Use common sense and professional medical advice.

Good body hygiene includes the following:

1. Wash your hands at the following times:

- Before eating anything
- After using any restroom, even your own
- After your hands are visibly soiled
- After handling pets, their food, or their bodily discards (loose hair, feces, urine, etc.)
- Anytime you come in skin contact with strangers, or those with an illness

- Before and while preparing foods
- When possible, after touching public access surfaces (such as subway hand rungs, escalator handrails, door handles, salad bar station tongs and utensils, the table at the food court at the mall, water fountains, grocery store carts, public telephones, the pen at the discount store everyone has used all day to sign credit card slips, gas station pumps, etc.)

2. Bathe daily.
3. Perform proper hair and nail care (fingers and toes).
4. Practice good oral care (daily flossing and tooth brushing, regular dental visits, etc.).
5. Practice good hygiene after using the restroom.
6. Keep a tube of germ jelly (antibacterial gel) with you, which can be used to help reduce surface bacteria.

SPECIAL NOTES ON YEAST INFECTIONS

A common yeast infection (Candida albicans) is defined as "misery" by anyone who has experienced one. Yeast will thrive in moist, unexposed areas of the body, especially the groin area, underarms, skin folds, and underneath the breasts of women.

To help prevent vaginal yeast infections:
1. Wear looser-fitting garments to allow air to circulate.
2. Wear all-cotton underwear.
3. Immediately dry off after showering, bathing, and swimming.
4. Cleanse and put on new garments if you become very sweaty.
5. Keep glucose levels in good control.
6. Practice good hygiene after using the restroom.
7. Talk to your doctor about yeast prevention measures (or possible medications) if you are prone to vaginal yeast infections, especially if you are prescribed a course of antibiotics, which may put you at higher risk of developing a yeast infection.

MAINTAIN A HEALTHY IMMUNE SYSTEM

- Reach and maintain a good level of physical fitness.
- Get good sleep each night.
- Do not smoke.

- Eat healthy, which includes seeking daily sources of vitamin C, protein, antioxidants, and other nutrients.
- Reduce stress.
- Keep bacteria from setting up camp inside your home. Keep kitchens and all areas where food is stored clean. Keep bathrooms clean, and keep pet food, hair, and waste away from you and your family.

MAINTAIN GOOD BLOOD GLUCOSE NUMBERS

- Check your blood glucose daily to see your numbers.
- Compare your numbers with your A1C level, at least quarterly.
- Comply with medical recommendations for your diabetes management plan, including the keys of a healthy meal plan, regular physical activity, and following medication treatment plans if prescribed.
- Don't be a stranger. Stay in contact with your health care providers. They should be able to know you by name rather than just the time of your appointment (for example, "Dr. Smith, your 11:30 is here to see you.").

TREAT MINOR PROBLEMS QUICKLY AND CORRECTLY

- Keep a basic first aid kit at your home, when your travel, and in your car (see Things to Know 34, "How to treat minor injuries")
- Become knowledgeable about over-the-counter products and remedies. Ask your health care professionals which ones are preferred products and which are not.
- Old remedies such as "putting butter on a burn," "sealing up a wound with a mud pack," "starve a cold and feed a fever," "just tough it out a few days," and others are not modern medical practices. Welcome the advances of the modern world.

USE COMMON SENSE AND PROFESSIONAL MEDICAL ADVICE

▌**Just call:** If you wonder if you should call about a problem, you probably should.

▌**Physician extenders: an extension of care:** Many physicians offer "nurse call" service, which allows your call about minor problems to be answered quickly by a trained nurse or health care professional.

▌**Free advice comes cheap:** Use the Internet cautiously. Some sites look great but may not have evidence-based medical advice.

▌**Is there a doctor in the house?** Just because the label on the product says "designed by a doctor," it doesn't mean the product is a good choice. Be a cautious consumer, and read before you buy.

▌**Lose the pointy toes, or you could lose your toes for good.** Choose footwear carefully. Buy good supportive shoes and breathable socks and hosiery items. Break in new shoes slowly, and check feet daily.

▌**Go to the bathroom when you need to. Don't be a hero.** Women and men can have urinary tract infections (also known as UTIs). Women, because of their anatomy, are at higher risk. To help prevent UTIs:

  ▌Drink plenty of fluids each day.
  ▌Empty your bladder at regular intervals.
  ▌Practice good hygiene after toileting and sexual intercourse.
  ▌Wear breathable underwear.

Note: Before taking herbal or nutritional treatments such as cranberry capsules or baby aspirin to prevent UTIs, talk to your physician first, since these remedies may create undesirable side effects when combined with other medications you are taking.

Finally, having diabetes complications such as neuropathy (nerve damage) and peripheral vascular disease (circulation problems) also contribute to a higher risk of infection. If you have either of these conditions, it is especially important to practice all infection prevention measures.

MORE RESOURCES TO EXPLORE

BOOKS

The Complete Guide to Diabetes, 4th edition. American Diabetes Association; Alexandria, VA, 2005.

WEBSITES

National Institutes of Health . . . . WWW.KIDNEY.NIDDK.NIH.GOV/
KUDISEASES/PUBS/UTIADULT
This section of the website for the National Institutes of Health, Kidney Disease deals specifically with urinary tract infections.

Women's Health . . . . HTTP://WWW.WOMENSHEALTH.GOV/
FAQ/VAGINAL-YEAST-INFECTIONS.CFM
This section of the Women's Health website, a division of the U.S. Department of Health and Human Services, gives information on yeast infections. This information is also available at 1-800-044-9662.

32
How to take care of illness

If you develop a problem, take a look at the provided chart that contains some tips on helping you take care of the issue. Keep in mind that being ill may cause your blood glucose to bounce around—no matter if the ailment is a minor ache or a full-blown case of the dreaded flu. Many people think if they don't eat normally, they don't need their diabetes medications. In fact, illness usually causes higher blood glucose levels. Make sure you have a sick-day plan worked out in advance from your health care professional. Always follow his or her professional advice. These general tips are meant for minor problems and are not meant to replace your physician's or health care provider's individualized instructions to you.

WAYS TO HELP AN ILLNESS

Problem	Tips
Fever	• Drink plenty of liquids. • Keep a fever thermometer available. • Know what type and how much fever-reducing medications to take. • Monitor blood glucose every 2–4 hours during a fever. • Take a tepid bath. • Check for ketones as directed by your health care provider. • Keep phone numbers handy in case you feel unable to care for yourself.
Head cold	• Drink plenty of liquids. • Use a humidifier or vaporizer to keep the air from being too dry. • Choose soft tissues to avoid skin irritation when wiping an overly runny nose. • Check with the pharmacist before using any over-the-counter cold product, and make sure the pharmacist knows the complete list of medications you are taking and your health conditions. • Ask questions before you buy products. • Get plenty of rest. • Don't push yourself—give yourself time to recover. • Check blood glucose levels every 4–6 hours while awake. • Don't smoke!
Sore throat	• Call your health care provider if you are unable to consume your regular meal plan. You may need to change your medicine if you are eating less, or you may need a change in food choices (perhaps by including some sugar-containing calorie boosters). • Call the doctor if the sore throat is accompanied by a fever or persists more than 2 days. • Use approved pain relievers (analgesics) for comfort. • Avoid sore-throat drops sold over the counter unless they are approved by your health care provider (they may contain hidden ingredients, including carbohydrates). • Drink plenty of fluids. • Rest your voice. • Check blood glucose levels every 4 hours while awake.

Problem	Tips
Sore throat (*continued*)	• Choose soft, non-spicy food if eating is painful. You may also need to eat smaller, more frequent meals to maintain your intake and avoid hypoglycemia. • Don't smoke!
Diarrhea	• Call your physician if you have had diarrhea for more than 4 hours. • Replace lost fluids by drinking clear, noncaffeinated liquids (water, diet soft drinks, diet powdered drinks, tea, etc.) every hour. • Avoid foods that may aggravate diarrhea (greasy foods, high-fiber foods, and sometimes dairy foods). • Choose bland foods such as baked meats, rice, plain potatoes, plain pasta, canned fruit, yogurt, artificially sweetened gelatin/puddings/popsicles, broth-based soups, crackers, and toast. • Check with a pharmacist before taking over-the-counter anti-diarrhea agents. • Try to eat small amounts every few hours. • Check for ketones if you have type 1 or are pregnant and your blood glucose level is staying above your target level.
Vomiting	• Call your physician if you have been vomiting for more than 4 hours. • Call your physician if you are unable to hold down liquids. • Call your physician if you cannot hold down foods for more than one meal (about 4 hours' duration). • Replace fluids by drinking room-temperature liquids. • If you can hold down fluids, but not solids, consume sugar-containing liquids or soft foods to provide calories and prevent hypoglycemia: regular gelatin, regular popsicles, apple or other transparent juices, frozen yogurt, sherbet, etc. • Slowly add in solids when you are more stable, such as plain crackers, toast (plain and unbuttered), dry cereal products, graham crackers, animal crackers, rice, mashed potatoes, etc. • Try to eat small amounts every few hours as you recover. • Call your physician if you have a fever. • Call your physician if you take premeal diabetes medications (pills or injections). You may need to change the amount or avoid them until your intake is back to normal.

Problem	Tips
Vomiting (*continued*)	• Call your physician if you have positive ketones or suspect diabetic ketoacidosis.
Flu/sinus or bronchial infection	• Notify your physician. • Get plenty of rest. • Drink fluids every hour. • Check blood glucose every 2–4 hours. • Check ketones as directed by your physician. • Ask the doctor if you may need supplemental insulin or a change in your medications to help control blood glucose. • Keep phone in reach, and have someone to contact if you are unable to care for yourself. • Notify your physician if you experience pain in your head, ears, chest, or abdomen. • Check your temperature every 2–4 hours. • Call your physician if you have positive ketones or suspect diabetic ketoacidosis. • Talk to your physician about an annual flu vaccination plan.
Abscess or draining wound	• Call your physician at once.

MORE RESOURCES TO EXPLORE

BOOKS

The Complete Guide to Diabetes, 4th edition. American Diabetes Association; Alexandria, VA. 2005.

WEBSITES

Bayer Health Care . . . . WWW.BAYERDIABETES.COM/US
   On the Bayer Health Care website you can find the document Sick-Day Management: Bayer Health Facts.

National Institutes of Health. . . . . HTTP://WWW.DIABETES.NIDDK.NIH.GOV/
   This is the website of the NIDDK, where you can find the document, "Taking Care of Your Diabetes At Special Times When You're Sick." You can also order a copy through the NIH at 1-800-860-8747.

33

What everyone should have in their medicine cabinet

Everyone should have a sick-day shelf with the following items in case of illness. Nothing is worse than feeling bad and not having the supplies you need in your apartment, dorm room, or house to give you relief or comfort. Plan ahead and keep important supplies and comforts available, because you just might wake up one morning feeling poorly.

Medication cabinets often become the storehouse for old toothbrushes, spare change, rusty razors, old prescriptions, and more. These items are not likely to be useful to you during an illness, and not even if you were in an extreme episode of a survival TV series on a desolate island in the ocean. Take a few extra minutes this weekend and see how your bathroom and kitchen cabinets measure up with this inventory list.

MUST HAVES

- ✓ Thermometer (a working one, and keep extra batteries on hand)
- ✓ Strips
- ✓ Analgesics/fever reducers (know which type is best for you—some people with kidney, liver, or heart problems may be limited to only certain types of these medications due to health conditions)
- ✓ Band-Aids
- ✓ Aloe vera gel or cream
- ✓ Antibiotic cream

- ✓ Antiseptic spray or liquid
- ✓ Gauze pads
- ✓ Ace bandage or wrap
- ✓ Ice pack (reusable freezer packs or frozen peas work well)
- ✓ Cortisone-based or anti-allergy skin cream
- ✓ Glucagon kit (if advised by your physician)
- ✓ Measuring spoons or medicine dispensing cups with increments clearly marked
- ✓ Ketone strips
- ✓ Paper and pencil for writing down blood glucose results, ketone results, temperature results, food intake, and new instructions from your health care professional
- ✓ A written plan on how to take care of yourself. It should include answers on:
  - ∎ What diabetes medications to take and not to take
    - ✓ Diabetes pills
    - ✓ Insulins
    - ✓ Other injectables (such as pramilitide, exenatide, etc.)
  - ∎ How often to check blood glucose levels
  - ∎ How often to check ketones
  - ∎ How much medication to take
  - ∎ What to eat
  - ∎ How to adjust pump settings (if on a pump)
  - ∎ When to call for help

FOODSTUFFS

- ✓ Regular and sugar-free sodas
- ✓ Regular and sugar-free gelatin and pudding mixes
- ✓ Regular and sugar-free popsicles
- ✓ Saltine crackers
- ✓ Canned low-fat, lower-sodium chicken or vegetable broth
- ✓ Peanut butter
- ✓ Individual containers of unsweetened applesauce
- ✓ Canned lite fruit

- ✓ Canned lower-sodium soups (both broth and cream based; get several small cans)
- ✓ Animal crackers or graham crackers
- ✓ Low-sugar sports drinks
- ✓ Instant mashed potatoes or rice
- ✓ Instant oatmeal, grits, or other cereal products
- ✓ Unsweetened juice that is shelf-stable at room temperature

OTHER ITEMS THAT ARE GOOD TO HAVE AROUND

- ✓ Extra gallons of drinking water
- ✓ Extra boxes of tissues
- ✓ Extra boxes of wipes
- ✓ Resealable plastic bags (for mini–ice pack relief)
- ✓ Small emergency cash supply, in case you need take a taxi, or to buy treatment items
- ✓ Short-acting insulin and syringes (if recommended by your health care professional), to treat acute hyperglycemia
- ✓ Health care professional–approved gastrointestinal remedies if you suffer from periodic digestive problems
- ✓ Disposable gloves
- ✓ Disinfectant spray and cleaners

THINGS TO GET RID OF

- ✓ Mercury / glass thermometers
- ✓ Expired prescriptions
- ✓ Expired over-the-counter medications
- ✓ Opened and "aged" items such as petroleum jellies, old lotions and creams, and gauze pads
- ✓ Expired ketone strips
- ✓ Expired glucagon kits
- ✓ Unknown containers of stuff

MORE RESOURCES TO EXPLORE

BOOKS

The Complete Guide to Diabetes, 4th edition. American Diabetes Association; Alexandria, VA, 2005.

WEBSITES

American Academy of Family
  Physicians . . . . HTTP://FAMILYDOCTOR.ORG
  This website for the American Academy of Family Physicians covers a variety of first aid tips.

American Diabetes Association . . . . WWW.DIABETES.ORG/YOUTHZONE/
  SURVIVING-SICK-DAYS.JSP
  This section of the American Diabetes Association website covers a number of sick-day tips and recommendations.

American Red Cross . . . . WWW.REDCROSS.ORG
  Website of the American Red Cross.

MedlinePlus . . . . WWW.NLM.NIH.GOV/MEDLINEPLUS/
  FIRSTAID.HTML
  Website for MedlinePlus, which brings together authoritative information from NLM, the National Institutes of Health, and other government agencies and health-related organizations. Pre-formulated MEDLINE searches are included in MedlinePlus and give easy access to medical journal articles. MedlinePlus also has extensive information about drugs, an illustrated medical encyclopedia, interactive patient tutorials, and the latest health news.

34

How to treat minor injuries

WHAT TO DO AND WHAT NOT TO DO WHEN TREATING MINOR INJURIES

Problem	What to do	What not to do	Other tips
Skin scrape or small cut	• Clean the area with soap and wash thoroughly. • Apply a small amount of antibiotic cream to the area. • Cover with a Band-Aid or gauze pad. • Call your doctor if the area does not progress in a day or two, or if it becomes inflamed (shows signs or puffiness, redness, and tenderness) or starts to drain or seep pus. • Change the Band-Aid or pad daily.	• Do not wipe the area with alcohol or iodine. • Do not purchase super-adhesive tapes and pads; they can cause further damage to the skin. • Do not pick at the scab or loose tissue; it will fall off when it is ready.	• For further protection, choose clothing the covers the area that was injured. • Keep 4 inch × 4 inch sterile gauze pads available for large wounds; ask your health care professional about safe tape to use on your skin.

Problem	What to do	What not to do	Other tips
Sunburn	• Apply aloe vera gel or a good quality moisturizing lotion several times a day. • Drink plenty of liquids. • Avoid the sun until the area heals.	• Do not take hot showers or long baths (they will cause further drying). • Do not go swimming (it will cause further drying). • Do not use petroleum jelly (it does not allow the skin to breathe well and may impede healing).	• Keep the area covered from further sun exposure. • Don't pick at peeling skin; it will slough off by itself.
Heat burn	• Immediately cool the affected area by using room-temperature or tepid water. • Apply aloe vera gel to the skin. • If the skin is broken or blisters immediately, seek medical care as soon as possible; you may have a second- or third-degree burn.	• Do not apply butter or mud packs; these old methods will hold in heat and cause further tissue damage. • Do not use ice water; it will further damage the tissue.	• Cover the area and protect it from exposure to sun and water as much as possible. • Sometimes a prescription medication may be needed, along with an antibiotic, if the burn is severe.

Problem	What to do	What not to do	Other tips
Blister on a heel	• Clean the area gently. • Cover with a protective pad and then call your health care provider to evaluate. • Get rid of the footwear that caused the problem.	• Do not let it go. • Do not continue to wear the same footwear that caused the damage. • Do not pop the blister with a pin or by squeezing.	• Evaluate your footwear for comfort each time you wear it. • Wear comfortable walking shoes if you are on your feet, or plan to travel.
Ingrown toenail	• Call your health care professional or see a podiatrist to treat. • Never try to perform bathroom surgery on yourself, especially your feet.	• Do not cut the toenail out yourself. • Do not wear tight shoes.	• Evaluate your footwear to make sure you are not contributing to the problem. • Practice proper foot care.
Toothache	• Call the dentist the first day you notice the symptoms. • Avoid hot and cold items. • Treat pain with a recommended analgesic product. • Keep blood glucose levels in good control to avoid an infection from starting.	• Do not apply heat packs to your cheek or jaw. • Do not let the toothache persist.	• Practice good oral hygiene. • Floss daily. • See dentist regularly.

Problem	What to do	What not to do	Other tips
Bee stings	• Remove the stinger gently if it is visible. • Seek medical attention if the stinger is not visible or is below the skin surface. • Cleanse the area and apply a small amount of an approved cortisone skin cream (check with your pharmacist).	• Do not use a mud pack. • Do not pick out the stinger with a sewing needle from home.	• Keep an approved cortisone cream on hand for insect bites, rashes, and stings.
Foreign body in the eye	• Try to flush out with clean warm water; if not successful, seek medical attention as soon as possible.	• Do not poke the surface of your eye with fingers (or someone else's) or use tweezers or other objects to remove a foreign body.	• Wear eye protection (goggles or glasses) when mowing, raking, painting, spraying, doing auto work, wood working, or performing any job with potentially flying debris.
Warts	• Call your health care provider or dermatologist as soon as you detect the wart.	• Do not try to cut the wart off or file it down yourself. • Do not treat with over-the-counter pads, drops, or creams.	• Wear water shoes in public showers. • Don't share footwear. • Spray shoes daily with a disinfectant spray during treatment of a wart to keep it from repeating.

Problem	What to do	What not to do	Other tips
Cracked, dry skin	• Take short baths and showers using tepid water. • Keep hydrated (drink plenty of fluids). • Use moisturizing soaps to cleanse. • Wear protective gloves when doing household cleaning, changing diapers, and gardening. • Gently pat the skin dry after showering and apply lotion. • Reapply lotion during the day when possible.	• Do not apply lotion or moisturizers between body folds (between toes, underarms, etc.). • Do not take long, hot showers or baths. • Do not wash dishes or clean the household barehanded. • Do not expose skin to extreme temperatures (hot or cold or wind). • Do not use lotions with a high alcohol content (read the label).	• Scratching can lead to an open wound. • Consider a home humidifier.

MORE RESOURCES TO EXPLORE

WEBSITES

American Academy of
Family Physicians. . . . . HTTP://FAMILYDOCTOR.ORG
This website for the American Academy of Family Physicians covers a variety of first aid tips.

American Red Cross. . . . . WWW.REDCROSS.ORG
Website of the American Red Cross.

MedlinePlus . . . . WWW.NLM.NIH.GOV/MEDLINEPLUS/
FIRSTAID.HTML
Website for MedlinePlus, which brings together authoritative information from NLM, the National Institutes of Health, and other government agencies and health-related organizations. Pre-formulated MEDLINE searches are included in MedlinePlus and give easy access to medical journal articles. MedlinePlus also has extensive information about drugs, an illustrated medical encyclopedia, interactive patient tutorials, and the latest health news.

35

How to plan for a baby

WHY SHOULD I PREPARE?

A fetus starts to develop right after conception. Waiting until you are already pregnant may be too late to prevent some problems. Good blood glucose control can reduce the risk of the following:

■ Miscarriage

■ Birth defects

■ Stillbirths

■ Macrosomia (large baby)

■ Premature delivery

■ Complications to both you and the unborn child during pregnancy and after birth

WHAT IS THE GOAL?

Blood glucose levels should be as close to normal as possible before conception and throughout pregnancy. This means you need to get "tight" with your control. Research has shown

Expected Date June 2nd

that higher numbers mean higher risk to both mom and the fetus.

PLANNING BEFORE GETTING PREGNANT

Is There Anything I Should Do Before I Get Pregnant, and How Far Out Should I Plan Because I Have Diabetes?

6 MONTHS BEFORE CONCEPTION

- Get a physical.
- Get an A1C check, and see how you are measuring up to your goal and to "normal."
- Review all your medications with your physician.
- Tell all your health care providers about your interest in becoming pregnant in the near future.
- Stop smoking.
- Stay on birth control until your physician feels your diabetes control is within desirable ranges.
- If you are worried about future weight gain because you are already overweight, meet with a registered dietitian now to lose the weight. Pregnancy is not a time to promote weight loss.
- Consider an insulin pump if you are on insulin. This device will allow you to perform frequent adjustments and truly fine-tune your insulin delivery, day and night!

3 MONTHS BEFORE CONCEPTION

- Get another A1C check.
- Talk to your diabetes health care professionals about what diabetes medications you should take during pregnancy. They will likely want you to switch to them now, which will help you "work out the kinks" in determining the right medication types and dosages for you before the fetus is conceived. If you were on "pills," your health care professionals may recommend you switch to insulin during the pregnancy, one reason being that insulin dosages and timing can be easily and quickly adjusted to fit your changing body's needs day by day.
- Research what OB/GYN you plan to use and make some phone calls to check on who your insurance covers and in which hospital you want

(continued)

to deliver, etc. Most OB/GYNs prefer a prepregnancy visit for new patients. Let them know you have diabetes. They may refer you to a doctor who specializes in high-risk pregnancies.

▪ Get a baseline eye exam by a trained ophthalmologist and again during the first and third trimesters of your pregnancy. Pregnancy can worsen eye problems, so get those peepers checked out.

▪ Fine-tune your meal plan—make sure you have a balanced intake of nutrients.

▪ Start on prescription prenatal vitamin/mineral supplements that contain folic acid, iron, and calcium.

▪ Avoid alcohol.

▪ Develop a good stress management plan.

▪ Stock up on testing supplies. You may need to test about four or more times a day now to help evaluate your control. Later in pregnancy, you can expect to test six to ten times a day. Best times to test are as follows:
  ▪ Fasting
  ▪ Before meals
  ▪ 1–2 hours after meals (check with your physician which is preferred)
  ▪ Bedtime
  ▪ Between 2:00 and 3:00 a.m.

▪ Get a medical ID if you don't already have one.

▪ Ask your diabetes health care professionals to "up" your prescriptions for lancets and strips now so you don't run out.

WHAT SHOULD YOU EXPECT WHEN YOU HAVE DIABETES AND YOU GET PREGNANT?

▪ Be prepared for lots of extra work. But it will be worth it to have a healthy child. Stay positive about what is being asked of you.

▪ Fluctuations in your blood glucose are not uncommon. Because of hormonal and metabolic changes in your body, your control will be changing at each stage of pregnancy. You may especially notice higher readings first thing in the morning because of the hormonal effects at night. Here are some other issues that may affect your blood glucose along the way:

- **First trimester (0–3 months):** Expect some possible hypoglycemia, especially if you experience morning sickness, nausea, or heartburn. Hypoglycemia may also occur as hormones begin to change.

- **Second trimester (3–6 months):** You have a greater need for calories to grow the fetus, which means you will be eating more and gaining weight. Thus, your need for diabetes medication will likely start to increase. The increase in weight is not only to grow the fetus, but to develop maternal fat stores. The higher body fat may also make your body more resistant to your own insulin or injected insulin, meaning frequent medication adjustments.

- **Third trimester (6–9 months):** Your activity may be less, and your weight will be steadily increasing. Pregnancy hormones are peaking now, and several make insulin less efficient in the body. For these three reasons, your need for medication may be twice as much as your prepregnancy medication needs (if you took it before). If you didn't already take diabetes medication, your doctor may need to start you now, even if you only have a few weeks to go.

- You should test your blood glucose levels more often.

- Expect daily ketone testing (using fasting, every morning).

- You'll change your medical nutrition plan. The same plan you consumed before will not be sufficient for calories and may have a different distribution of carbohydrate than before. A typical meal plan for pregnancy will have the following:

  - Six small meals a day, rather than three large ones
  - Less carbohydrate at breakfast
  - A different balance of carbohydrate, protein, and fat
  - Allowances for calcium-rich foods
  - Limitations on fish and seafood, which may contain mercury
  - High-fiber foods to aid digestion (pregnancy can cause constipation)
  - Nutrient-dense foods (healthy choices)

■ Prepare for unexpected swings.

  ■ Always carry low blood glucose treatments with you.

  ■ Perform frequent testing to catch problems before they get out of hand.

  ■ Supplemental insulin injections may be needed to treat "highs."

■ You'll need encouragement to stay active. Keeping your body healthy will help you control your blood glucose as well as keep you in good shape. There are good prenatal exercise classes at many types of facilities: hospitals, local fitness centers, yoga centers, and health departments. Ask your OB/GYN about what is safe and best for you and your body.

■ Make regular visits to your OB/GYN and diabetes health care provider.

■ Be open-minded to breast-feeding—read about it.

■ Practice self-management.

■ Get all the rest you can—you are going to need it!

MORE RESOURCES TO EXPLORE

BOOKS

101 Tips for a Healthy Pregnancy with Diabetes, by Patti Geil and Laura Heironymus. American Diabetes Association; Alexandria, VA, 2003.

Diabetes and Pregnancy: What to Expect, 4th edition. American Diabetes Association; Alexandria, VA, 2001.

WEBSITES

Centers for Disease Control . . . . WWW.CDC.GOV/NCBDDD/BD/DIABETESPREGNANCYFAQS.HTM
  This is a section of the Centers for Disease Control and Prevention, Department of Health and Human Services website, titled "Diabetes and Pregnancy: Frequently Asked Questions."

Diabetic Mommy . . . . WWW.DIABETICMOMMY.COM
  The website for Diabetic Mommy, an online magazine.

March of Dimes. . . . . WWW.MARCHOFDIMES.COM

CHAPTER 8

PREVENT PROBLEMS DOWN THE ROAD

36

Ten things to do for those 10 toes

1. **Look.** Look at your feet and toes every day. Don't forget to check between piggy number two and piggy number three, and so on. Use a hand mirror to help you if need be.

2. **Stop smoking.** Smoking causes poor circulation and therefore puts you at higher risk of complications if you have an injury to your foot. Damage is taking place on the inside of the foot from smoking, affecting the circulation. An external injury will create two difficult problems to treat.

3. **Get up.** Whether you choose to garden outside, dance in the kitchen, walk with friends at a mall, or any other physical activity, body movement on a regular basis will help your overall circulation and muscle tone.

4. **Think features before fashion.** Choose footwear carefully. Look for comfortably fitting shoes, and inspect the quality of materials used to make the product. Break in all shoes gradually.

5. **Take 15 minutes to check your sock drawer.** Get rid of all the lone rangers (whose partners got eaten by the dryer), those with "un-elastic" elastic, those with superpower-mark-leaving elastic, "Sunday" socks (holey socks!), and any others that cause irritation. Pitch the nylon ones or those that keep in perspiration. Excess perspiration on your toes can lead to bacterial and fungal growth, as well as contribute to stinky feet.

6. **Wiggle those toes while you wait.** If you must sit for long periods of time, try to move your toes periodically, as well as try to

do some "seated dancing" or aerobics under the desk or table to keep the blood pumping around. Try *not* to cross your legs or ankles—that will further restrict circulation. For comfort, move one foot slightly in front of the other rather than crossing them.

7. **Soap and water.** Wash your feet daily in warm soapy water. Keep your feet clean, dry, and protected each day. **Do not go barefoot.** Practice safe nail care or see a podiatrist if you cannot safely perform this action. Use caution at nail salons—make sure they are following all local health and safety requirements to avoid getting a problem from a previous customer, such as nail fungal infections or plantar warts.

8. **Moisturize.** Your skin is your feet's first and best defense against the hazards of the world. Keep your "armor" in good condition by using a daily moisturizer, but don't apply it between the toes. Use a pumice stone to gently keep calluses down. Report any breaks in the skin to a health care provider to evaluate. Drinking lots of liquids will also help keep your skin supple.

9. **Not your favorite thing to do?** Ask your health care professional to take a good long look at your precious feet at each visit. It might not be your favorite thing to do, but it could prevent problems in the end. Swallow your pride. Remember it isn't a beauty contest—it's a matter of your health. Aren't your feet worth keeping?

10. **Love those feet.** Make it a priority to practice good foot care every day. You only get one body and one set to work with—don't abuse them.

MORE RESOURCES TO EXPLORE

BOOKS

101 Tips on Foot Care for People with Diabetes, 2nd edition, by Jessie H. Ahroni and Neil M. Scheffler. American Diabetes Association; Alexandria, VA, 2005.

37

How to take care of painful or numb feet

WHAT IS NEUROPATHY?

Neuropathy, or nerve damage, is one of the chronic complications of diabetes. Nerve damage can change the way a body part functions and its structure. People with type 1 or type 2 diabetes can develop this problem, and it can be difficult to treat. The cause of neuropathy isn't always clear when comparing "who gets it" and "who doesn't get it." Some factors may make you more prone to develop this condition. Factors that you cannot change, such as genetics and other health conditions, influence whether you may be at higher risk for neuropathy. The good news is there are some risk factors you can change to lower your risk, such as smoking (stop!), being overweight (try to achieve a desirable body weight), and controlling your blood glucose (watch your A1C levels to see how you are doing).

WHEN DOES NEUROPATHY START?

There is no set time frame of when nerve damage will appear. It is associated with blood glucose levels staying high for long periods of time. Sometimes nerve damage will happen without any symptoms, but then a person may start to notice some changes in a particular area of the body. Usually, the feet are affected first. This is called peripheral neuropathy. Nerve damage in the feet can affect how the foot moves, its shape, and its sensations (how the foot feels). The person who is beginning to develop neuropathy may first experience some "tingling" or "prickly" sensations periodically, especially at night. At the first sign of changes in your feet, seek medical attention. If you perform daily foot checks, you will be practicing good preventative screening each day and be alerted to any early signs of neuropathy.

If the damage progresses, numbness or pain becomes more prevalent. Some common symptoms of neuropathy in the feet and legs are:

▌Burning sensations
▌Stinging sensations
▌Tingling
▌Sharp pain
▌Stabbing sensations in a localized area
▌Crawling skin
▌High sensitivity to touch (bed sheets can cause pain)
▌Numbness
▌"Pins and needles" sensations

Pain is usually the first sign, but not the most dangerous symptom. When numbness occurs, it is signaling that your natural reactions to sensation are blocked, including reactions to a painful stimulus such as stepping on something sharp. Normally, when you step on something painful (hot or sharp or irritating), you instantly feel it and have a reaction to pull your foot away. Without this defense, you could incur a serious injury to your feet.

A common reason for amputation of the toe, foot, or leg is an initial injury caused by a lack of feeling by the person. A traumatic injury to the foot is hard to heal to begin with because of circulation issues (the feet are the farthest part away from your beating heart), but adding diabetes will also increase the risk of infection or poor healing. Ideally, at the first sign of an injury to a foot or leg, the person with diabetes should seek medical attention. Please see the box for some common injuries and prevention measures to use to help prevent traumatic injuries to the feet.

COMMON INJURIES AND HOW TO PREVENT THEM

Common injury	Prevention
Burns to the feet	▮ Never step into a jacuzzi, hot tub, or bath without carefully checking the temperature first (with elbow or thermometers).
	▮ Don't walk barefoot ever, but especially on a beach, boat, or pool area; these areas can be blistering hot.
	▮ Wear footwear that covers the entire foot, such as water shoes for summer water activities; and wear indoor house shoes or regular shoes when doing household chores.
Cuts to the feet	▮ Always check your shoes with your hand before stepping into your shoes.
	▮ Perform regular and proper nail care.
	▮ Never use nail scissors or blades on your feet.
Calluses/ blisters	▮ Choose properly fitting shoes.
	▮ Wear appropriate socks.
	▮ Wear the appropriate shoe for the right activity (walking shoes for travel, supportive shoes for those who work standing for long periods of time, etc.).

WHAT ARE TREATMENTS FOR NEUROPATHY?

To relieve pain, prevent further damage, and protect the feet, physical therapy and exercise can be performed or the patient can undergo the following treatments:

▮ Nerve stimulation—An external device is used to deliver electrical stimulation to relieve pain.

▮ Anodyne treatments—A noninvasive method that uses infrared light to stimulate nerve function.

▮ Massage—Rhythmic, gentle touches by hand or small devices to help with pain management, anxiety, and help to increase relaxation.

▮ Acupuncture:—Non-pharmaceutical method using thin needles that penetrate the skin to help restore "harmony" in the body as well as reduce pain.

- Biofeedback—An alternative medicine method using counseling to teach a person to train their body's responses and reaction to pain, to lessen the severity.
- Others—Complementary medicine practices, nutritional supplements, herbal remedies, counseling.

Also, medications such as pain relievers, antidepressants (these drugs seem to have a positive effect on symptoms), neuropathy medications, and topical creams are available. Some patients are fitted by their podiatrist for aids such as orthotics for shoes (from a podiatrist or orthotics specialist), braces, and custom shoes. Nutritional supplements may also be recommended, such as anti-oxidants (including alpha lipoic acid and others). Before taking any nutritional supplement, check with your physician. A reliable source for nutritional supplements and their uses can be found at the website for the National Center for Complementary and Alternative Medicine site (see More Resources to Explore).

WHAT CAN RESULT FROM NEUROPATHY?

Because of the changes in nerve function, structural problems can occur. Some common secondary problems from neuropathy include:

- Hammertoes
- Toe alignment problems
- Charcot foot (weakened bones, resulting in changes in the shape of the foot to where the foot has a "rocker bottom" structure)
- Gait problems (walking differently because of painful or numb feet)
- Lower back problems from walking improperly

WHAT CAN YOU DO TO KEEP NEUROPATHY FROM GETTING WORSE?

- Keep a close eye on your feet—check them daily.
- Follow medical advice to take care of your body and your diabetes.
- Report any problems or notable changes in your body functions at once to a qualified health care professional.
- Keep your blood glucose in a good range.
- If you are dealing with chronic pain, ask for information on

medical treatment as well as coping with chronic pain—depression is common in those with chronic pain.

❚ Learn about new treatments and support groups from local and national resources (see More Resources to Explore, below).

Caution

Don't let just anyone advise you or treat your feet if you have been diagnosed with neuropathy. Seek out a qualified health care professional, such as an endocrinologist, orthopedic doctor, or podiatrist.

MORE RESOURCES TO EXPLORE

BOOKS

Uncomplicated Guide to Diabetes Complications, 3rd edition, by Marvin Levin and Michael Pfeifer. American Diabetes Association; Alexandria, VA, 2009.

American Diabetes Association Guide to Herbs and Nutritional Supplements, by Laura Shane-McWhorter. American Diabetes Association; Alexandria, VA, 2009.

WEBSITES

American Chronic Pain Association . . . . HTTP://WWTHEACPA.ORG
  Website of the American Chronic Pain Association.

American College of Foot and
  Ankle Surgeons . . . . WWW.FOOTPHYSICIANS.COM
  Website of the American College of Foot and Ankle Surgeons.

dLife. . . . . WWW.DLIFE.COM
  Website of dLife, which contains information on peripheral neuropathy, amputation support, and Medicare shoe benefits.

National Institute of Neurological
  Disorders and Stroke. . . . . WWW.NINDS.NIH.GOV
  Website of the National Institute of Neurological Disorders and Stroke.

Neuropathy Association . . . . WWW.NEUROPATHY.ORG
  Website of the Neuropathy Association.

National Center for Complementary
  and Alternative Medicine . . . . HTTP://NCCAM.NIH.GOV/HEALTH/
                                                                    DIABETES/CAM-AND-DIABETES.HTM
  Website of National Center for Complementary and Alternative Medicine.

38

Sensible things to take care of your senses

YOUR EYES: HOW YOU SEE THE WORLD

WHAT PART OF THE EYE IS AFFECTED BY DIABETES?

Diabetes can cause damage to five parts of your eye:

■ Retina: The tissue in the back of the eye that transmits visual images received by the eye to the brain through the optic nerve

■ Vitreous: The clear matter within the eye between the lens and the retina

■ Lens: The front of eye that brings in light and images

■ Optic nerve: The largest nerve of the eye, it carries visual images by way of electric impulses from the retina to the brain

■ Blood vessels: These carry blood to your eye and can get clogged, just like other vessels

HOW IS THE EYE AFFECTED?

High glucose and high blood pressure are factors that can contribute to higher risk of eye disease and complications. The blood vessels in the eye are very tiny and fragile. Changes in the bloodstream components and blood pressure can weaken or damage the vessels and structures within the eye. Glaucoma, cataracts, retinopathy, and macular degeneration are eye problems seen in people with diabetes.

■ **Glaucoma:** Glaucoma is a common eye problem in people with diabetes. It results from having increased pressure in the eye and negatively affects the optic nerve functions. Individuals may or may not have symptoms at its onset but may experience occasional eye pain.

- **Cataracts:** Cataracts describe a condition when the lens of the eye changes from clear to cloudy. Individuals may experience night vision problems and sensitivity to bright light.
- **Retinopathy:** Retinopathy describes a progressive eye disease affecting the blood vessels in the eye. There are various stages of retinopathy. Some common symptoms are "seeing black spots." Early intervention can slow the progression of this disease.
- **Macular degeneration:** Macular degeneration refers to the damage caused in the central part of the retina and directly affects visual ability. The damage is usually noticed by an individual when central vision is not as good as "side" vision.

WHAT SHOULD YOU DO TO TAKE CARE OF YOUR EYES?

Get an annual eye examination. The eye exam should include the following:

- Vision screening (how well you can see/read)
- Glaucoma test (measures the "pressure" of your eye using tonometry, a special tool, or other techniques)
- Slit lamp (a special magnifying microscope used to see inside your eye; your eyes may be dilated first)
- Retinal scan (to see in the back of your eye; can be performed by high-tech cameras and other instruments)
- Cataract exam (a slit lamp is often used to see if the lens is becoming cloudy)
- Color vision exam (to see how you discern colors)

WHO SHOULD YOU SEE?

Know the differences among eye care professionals. Ideally, individuals with diabetes should see a qualified ophthalmologist.

What is an optometrist? An optometrist is a professional who has achieved the degree of doctor of optometry (OD) and who specializes in vision problems with glasses, contacts, and other aids. They can prescribe eye wear, certain aids, and medications to treat eye problems.

What is an optician? An optician is a professional who makes and/or sells eyewear (glasses or contacts), based on prescriptions received from a qualified optometrist or ophthalmologist.

What is an ophthalmologist? An ophthalmologist is a medical doctor (MD) who specializes in the diagnosis and treatment of eye problems (not just vision), including treatment of chronic eye conditions and disease. These professionals are qualified to also perform medical and surgical procedures related to eye treatment and care.

Note: There are civic organizations (Lions Club International, for example), as well as professional organizations (American Academy of Ophthalmology), who can help you find a qualified health care provider for eye care in your area. These organizations also help with reduced-cost or free exams in many situations and areas of the country for those who cannot afford care.

WHAT SHOULD YOU TAKE TO YOUR APPOINTMENT?

▮ Bring your glasses or contacts.
▮ Know your family health history, especially any eye problems.
▮ Bring a list of your current medications.
▮ Have questions ready about vision changes.
▮ Bring a pair of sunglasses (in case they dilate your eye).

WHAT IS THE BEST DEFENSE FOR EYE DISEASE?

Early detection is the best defense! Get your annual eye exams, even if you are seeing well.

YOUR MOUTH: A SMILE IS WORTH ITS WEIGHT IN GOLD

HOW IS YOUR MOUTH AFFECTED BY DIABETES?

Diabetes increases the incidence of several mouth problems, including increased plaque (the sticky film of bacteria that develops on your teeth), fungal infections, taste impairment, and periodontal disease (gum disease). Poor hygiene or excess bacteria can also cause bad breath and frequent canker sores.

High glucose in the bloodstream means higher amounts of glucose in your saliva. Saliva is present in your mouth and contains a certain amount of bacteria. Bacteria can grow more quickly with "more food" (glucose) around, and problems with plaque occur more frequently in people with diabetes.

WHAT SHOULD YOU DO TO TAKE CARE OF YOUR MOUTH?

- Brush your teeth twice a day (when rising and before bedtime).
- Floss daily between all teeth.
- Take care of mouth appliances.

HOW TO PROPERLY BRUSH YOUR TEETH

1. Find out what type of toothbrush is best for you. You may be surprised to find out that your dentist recommends a "soft" brush. These soft bristles can remove plaque very well, provided you put in enough time at the sink. Extra-firm bristles might be abrasive to your tender gum line, or cause friction and possible localized abrasions or ulcers.

2. It is more time, not more force, that produces good results. Aim for about 1 minute for the top and 1 minute for the bottom set of teeth.

3. Choose the proper toothpaste. Look for fluoride content, not Hollywood smile promises.

4. Think dimensional. Teeth have a top, front sides, back sides, and shared space with their neighbor tooth. Clean all these sides well each time you brush.

5. Clean dental plates, partials, bite guards, and other mouth appliances daily as directed.

6. Choose flossers that allow you to get all the way down to the gum line. Have an expert (a dental hygienist or dentist) show you how it's done and recommend a product for you.

7. Change your toothbrush often, especially after viral or bacterial illnesses.

8. If you have a problem with cavities, ask about prescription toothpastes or rinses that contain higher levels of fluoride, which is proven to fight cavities.

- Contact your dentist if your gums are tender, swollen, red, or bleed easily.
- Contact your doctor if you have persistent bad breath or taste impairment.

WHO SHOULD YOU SEE?

See your dentist twice a year. A dental hygienist may clean your teeth, but you need a qualified dentist to evaluate your mouth. Let your dentist know you have diabetes.

WHAT ELSE CAN I DO TO TAKE CARE OF MY MOUTH AND TEETH?

- Choose a wide variety of crunchable and chewy foods that allow you to practice good chewing (fiber-rich foods such as fruits and vegetables).
- Don't smoke.
- Keep blood glucose levels in a good range.
- Eat a healthy diet.
- Don't share lipsticks, lip makeup, or chapsticks.
- If you can't brush after a meal, at least rinse your mouth with water.

WHAT IS THE BEST DEFENSE?

Preventative daily oral care is the best defense. Keep those pearly whites clean!

YOUR NERVOUS SYSTEM: SENSATIONS

HOW IS YOUR NERVOUS SYSTEM AFFECTED BY DIABETES?

Neuropathy is a common diabetes complication that results in changes in your nervous system. Your nervous system is made up of specialized nerve cells that perform many body functions. Not only do nerve cells allow us to "feel," but they help control functions of the body as well.

Nerves help with the following:

- How your stomach empties
- How your bladder empties
- Sexual functions

- How your intestines function
- How your body responses to various needs
- How your body reacts to stimulus (good ones such as touch and bad ones such as stepping on a sharp object)
- How muscles work

WHAT SHOULD YOU DO TO TAKE CARE OF YOUR NERVOUS SYSTEM?

- Perform daily foot exams to detect any early signs of numbness or pain in your feet.
- Get annual exams (full exams), not just looking over your A1C. Nerves are all over your body, controlling many systems.
- Take an active role in being an advocate for your body. Report any changes in body functions to your health care professional early.
- Don't be afraid to ask questions about sensitive issues, such as toileting and sexual function. Your health care professional will treat these issues professionally and confidentially.

WHO SHOULD YOU SEE?

See your health care professional regularly.

WHAT IS THE BEST DEFENSE?

Thorough annual exams are the best defense!

OTHER PROACTIVE HEALTH STEPS YOU CAN TAKE

1. Ask your doctor about an annual flu shot.
2. Ask your doctor if you should consider having a pneumonia vaccine.
3. Ask your doctor if you should have tetanus vaccine.
4. Ask your doctor about hepatitis B vaccines.
5. Women should keep appointments with their OB/GYN for annual exams.

MORE RESOURCES TO EXPLORE

WEBSITES

American Dental Association . . . . .WWW.ADA.ORG
Website of the American Dental Association.

American Academy of Ophthalmology . . .WWW.AAO.ORG
Foundation of the American Academy of Ophthalmology.

American Academy of Ophthalmology:
Glossary. . . . . .WWW.AAO.ORG/EYECARE/GLOSSARY
This section of the American Academy of Ophthalmology website contains a glossary of eye-related terms.

Lions Club International . . . . .WWW.LIONSCLUB.ORG
Website for Lions Club International.

National Diabetes Information
Clearinghouse .WWW.DIABETES.NIDDK.NIH.GOV
Website for the National Diabetes Information Clearinghouse, where you can find the documents Keep Your Diabetes Under Control and Keep Your Eyes Healthy.

39

How to reduce your risk of a heart attack

By now you know that lifestyle factors such as eating right, not smoking, and staying active will help you reduce your risk of a heart attack. Here are some other tips to help you avoid the number one complication of diabetes.

BEST CHOICES FOR YOUR PANTRY AND REFRIGERATOR

- ✓ Nonfat dairy products
- ✓ Fish (twice a week)
- ✓ Lean and extra-lean meat
- ✓ Plenty of fresh fruits and vegetables
- ✓ Nuts
- ✓ Whole-grain products
- ✓ Monounsaturated oils such as canola, peanut, or olive
- ✓ Polyunsaturated oils such as safflower and sunflower
- ✓ Dried beans and legumes
- ✓ Salt-free seasonings (e.g., herbs and spices, low-sodium condiments)
- ✓ Lower-fat and -sodium soups and prepared foods
- ✓ Egg substitutes
- ✓ Trans-fat–free, low-calorie margarine
- ✓ Vegetable cooking spray
- ✓ Low-fat snacks such as light popcorn, baked chips, artificially sweetened popsicles, etc.

> **TIP:** Take a few minutes to inventory your pantry. Then change out items each week as you shop, and make food changes slowly for a more accepting transition.

WHAT ABOUT ALCOHOL?

Recommendations have changed about alcohol and what type may be beneficial or not. There are many ongoing studies evaluating if certain types of alcohol, such as red wine, have a beneficial effect in preventing heart disease in the general population. Red wine has special components known as antioxidants and flavonoids from the grapes from which it was produced. Red wine has been under the microscope for years, because of famous studies showing some European and Mediterranean countries' diets and their lower rates of heart disease. One factor that came out of these studies was the intake of red wine in the populations. But in recent years, caution has been taken about the findings. The medical researchers feel other factors play a role, such as genetics, smoking, diet composition, exercise, and other lifestyle factors that could have affected the outcomes. It has also been shown that too much alcohol intake increases the amount of triglycerides in the blood—another type of fat that causes damage as well.

SO WHAT IS THE FINAL WORD?

For now, the medical community feels drinking more than moderate levels (one glass for a woman, two glasses for a man per day) not only may elevate triglycerides, but may nullify the benefits of alcohol associated with heart disease prevention.

> **TIP:** Until more evidence is analyzed, if you do drink, drink in moderation only (one glass for a woman, two for a man) per day. Tell your health care professional if you consume alcohol on a regular basis.

WHAT'S A SERVING?

Serving sizes are 12 oz of beer, 5 oz of wine, and 1 1/2 oz of hard liquor.

WHAT ABOUT ASPIRIN THERAPY?

For individuals who have significant heart disease risk factors (positive family history, obesity, hypertension, smoking, and are over 40 years of age), your health care professional may recommend a daily low dose of aspirin. Aspirin is an anticoagulant (blood thinner) and has been shown in research to decrease the risk of heart attacks and strokes in people with diabetes. People who are aspiring sensitive or who suffer from certain health conditions (bleeding ulcers, or are on anticoagulation therapy already) may be prescribed alternative medications.

TIP: Ask your doctor if aspirin therapy is advised for you. Never start on medications on your own. Check with your doctor to avoid possible drug interactions or unfortunate side effects.

HOW MUCH IS A LOW DOSE?

A low dose is 75- to 162-mg tablets.

WHAT ABOUT NUTRIENT SUPPLEMENTS? WHO DO YOU BELIEVE?

The best way for you to get the daily nutrients you need is by eating a healthy diet. There are magazines filled with recommendations encouraging individuals to take extra amounts of vitamins, minerals, and other nutrients and compounds as prevention.

The United States Department of Agriculture (USDA) has many evidenced-based scientific studies that help to create the recommendations for vitamins and minerals. You have seen this information if you look at a food label, in terms of how much of a nutrient it provides compared with the USDA standards. There have been times when the recommenda-

TIP: Ask a qualified health care professional about nutritional supplements and the claims before investing your money. Some supplements may also interfere with your current medications, so once again, wait before you take.

tions have changed, based on strong clear evidence from research. As you read a claim, look to see if a trusted, known, scientific agency is making the recommendation, or if it is just an individual or a profit-making company.

WHAT ABOUT FISH OIL?

The American Heart Association has recommended that Americans eat a variety of fish twice a week as a preventative measure against heart disease. The types of fish recommended contain omega-3 fatty acids, which are components shown to have beneficial effects for those at risk of, or who have, heart disease. Omega-3 fatty acids can also be made from other nutrient forms (precursors); therefore, you may see claims about non-fish sources, too.

Omega-3 fatty acids can be found in mackerel, lake trout, herring, sardines, salmon, albacore tuna, tofu, soybeans, canola oil, walnuts, flaxseed, and other sources.

Do some types of fish contain mercury? Unfortunately, we have polluted the waters of the world so much, that yes, many of the abovementioned cold water fish are affected by mercury poisoning from pollution. For that reason, it is wise to consume fish in modest amounts, such as twice a week as described (a serving is 4–6 oz). The highest sources of mercury come from shark, swordfish, king mackerel, and tilefish. The U.S. Department of Health and Human Services and the Environmental Protection Agency have specific guidelines for women who might become pregnant, who are pregnant or nursing, and children.

BRUSH AND FLOSS YOUR TEETH

People with gum disease have a much higher rate of heart disease and stroke, according to the American Academy of Periodontology (study of gums). There are research studies that show a link, but why? One theory is, if gum disease is present, the inflammation of the blood vessels make them vulnerable to problems. Another theory points the blame at the extra bacteria in the blood, perhaps allowing more opportunity for plaque (causes narrowing of the blood vessels and blockages), within the blood vessels. Because of this, make extra effort to perform good daily mouth care and see a dentist regularly.

> **TIP:** 2-1-6 are numbers to remember: Brush twice, floss once, and see the dentist every 6 months.

KNOW YOUR NUMBERS: WHAT'S THE GOAL?

There is no number that is perfect for everyone. Each individual will need to work with their health care team to determine what goals are best for them. Following are the general recommendations of the American Diabetes Association.

	Goal	Reason
A1C	<7%	High levels of glucose in the blood have been shown to increase blood vessel damage, especially in individuals whose blood glucose has been elevated for 3 months.
Triglycerides	<150 mg/dl	High triglycerides are associated with blood vessel damage and are usually higher in people who consume alcohol or processed sweet/fatty foods.
LDL (low-density lipoproteins, part of a cholesterol profile)	<100 mg/dl	These are sticky fats that cause buildup blockages in blood vessels and are usually higher in people who consume saturated fats and cholesterol.
HDL (high-density lipoproteins, part of a cholesterol profile)	>40 mg/dl for men and >50 mg/dl for women	These are "helping" fats that may help keep blood vessels clean and are usually higher in people who are physically active.
Blood pressure	130/80 mmHg (Check with your doctor; this may be individualized)	High blood pressure puts more strain on the heart.
BMI (body mass index)	<25	BMI measures your body fat in relation to your overall body weight; being overweight or obese increases your chance of a heart attack and stroke.
Goal weight	This is always individualized, but you will probably be asked to lose 10% of your body weight if you are diagnosed with type 2 diabetes	Know what your desirable body weight is. If you are not at target, talk to your health care provider regarding weight loss plans.

MORE RESOURCES TO EXPLORE

WEBSITES

American Academy of Periodontology ..... WWW.PERI.ORG
   Website of the American Academy of Periodontology.

American Diabetes Association .... WWW.DIABETES.ORG
   Website of the American Diabetes Association. Be sure to check out the Make the Link! Diabetes, Heart Disease, and Stroke section of the website.

Institute of Medicine .... WWW.IOM.EDU
   Website of the Institute of Medicine, which contains information on vitamins and minerals, recommended nutrient intake.

Food and Drug Administration............ WWW.CFSAN.FDA.GOV
   Here you can find the free brochure "Mercury in Fish and Shellfish."

USDA National Agriculture Library........ HTTP://FNIC.NAL.USDA.GOV
   Website of the U.S. Department of Agriculture, National Agriculture Library, which contains information on vitamins, minerals, and recommended nutrient intake.

How to keep your love life happy

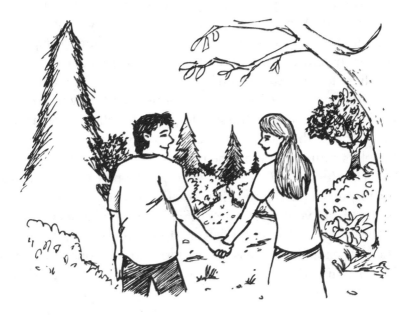

Diabetes can affect your love life emotionally (lack of sex drive) and physically (sexual dysfunction). Here are some issues related to sexual health. See if you know the correct answer to these 10 true or false questions.

1. The doctor will regularly ask me about my health, so I can just wait for him or her to bring up the subject.
   FALSE
   You will need to be the one to bring issues about your body to the attention of your health care professional. It may be uncom-

fortable, and you might not know all the medical terms to use to describe a situation, but communicate with your health care professional about changes in your love life. If it helps, write it down in a note. Changes in interest or physical changes related to sexual function may be related to your diabetes and can be addressed—that is, if the health care professional knows about it.

2. Sexual history is not a significant part of my medical history, so I shouldn't waste the doctor's time. It's my problem.
   FALSE

Sexual history is part of your medical history and well-being. It is a part of your private life and may be difficult to bring up. It is important for this part of your life to be discussed. Diabetes can cause physical changes in all parts of your body. People of any age should communicate issues with their doctors. The professionals in your doctor's office are not going to judge you. They are there to help. Some men believe they will be considered "a dirty old man" for bringing it up—this is certainly not the case. And if you are female and would prefer to talk to a female about the problem, then ask for a referral. You may wish to talk to just the physician rather than the person at the front desk about the problem. Just tell them you have a specific private question to ask the physician during the visit. You deserve to receive privacy and respect from your physician's office. If you do not feel your doctor or the staff makes you feel comfortable about a personal issue such as sexual health, ask for a referral to someone else. You need to feel comfortable with whoever provides you with guidance and treatment.

3. My problem must be diabetes related. I guess I will just have to live with it.
   FALSE

Find out if the problems you are having may be related to other causes, such as genito-urinary infections, a side effect from a medication, a vaginal infection, stress, or depression. Your doctor may refer you to a urologist or an OB/GYN who has specialty training in urinary and reproductive body systems.

4. Only men have problems with sexual dysfunction.

FALSE

Females can experience complications related to sexual function with diabetes, too, although they are generally less likely to talk about it. Changes can be related to an individual's sex drive, as well as physical changes. Males and females can experience sexual dysfunction at any time during their adult life, or into their geriatric years. Women should keep up with annual OB/GYN exams, as well as report changes if they occur. Sometimes in women, there are other factors that may contribute to sexual dysfunction, including menopause changes, hormone imbalances, and other issues.

5. If I already have problems, keeping my blood glucose down isn't going to help anything.

FALSE

High blood glucose will likely cause more damage to occur. In addition, in the short term, high blood glucose levels can contribute to bladder and vaginal infections, which can compound problems. Stay aggressive with blood glucose control even if you have experienced some diabetes complications. You never know when a new treatment may be just around the corner, and treatments are usually the most effective when complications are on a milder level, versus on a more serious level.

6. I can just quit taking my blood pressure medications because I heard some can cause sexual problems.

FALSE

Treat your high blood pressure. It can save your life. It is true—some blood pressure medications (and some other types of medications) may actually contribute to erectile dysfunction in men. Instead of not taking them, discuss options with your health care professional to find one that works best for you. Ask the pharmacist about side effects with any new prescription you get. Be informed.

7. Sexual performance problems are all in your head.

FALSE

There are many causes of sexual dysfunction, including both mental and physical issues. It is true that anxiety and stress can contribute to sexual dysfunction. Counseling can be helpful to discuss emotions and to help reduce stress, anxiety, and troubling concerns. Counseling can also be helpful if you are going through physical treatment of sexual dysfunction, to address your feelings about this sensitive aspect of your life.

8. Vaginal dryness is considered a sexual dysfunction.

TRUE

Vaginal dryness can cause irritation and pain during sex, thus contributing to a lack of interest in sex. Find out about medications that are available to help with dryness and irritation. Get recommendations. Do not just buy medications off the shelf, since some may not be good choices, or you may need detailed instruction on their use. There are also effective prescription medications available.

9. Avoiding tobacco may help treat sexual dysfunction.

TRUE

Tobacco products can cause further damage to blood vessels. The blood vessels in our sexual organs are fragile and could be damaged internally by high blood pressure, high blood glucose, and intake of tobacco and excessive intake of alcohol. The damage can affect how the body parts function. Smokers should stop smoking. If you drink, keep your alcohol consumption to the recommended amounts.

10. Drug treatments are the only options for treating sexual dysfunction.

FALSE

Counseling, devices, and other treatments can be used for treating sexual dysfunction. Ask about what treatments might be right for you. Learn more about treatments from trained experts, not grocery store magazine ads. Seek out a urologist (for men) or a gynecologist (for women) to get the most up-to-date information.

MORE RESOURCES TO EXPLORE

BOOKS

Sex and Diabetes: For Him and For Her, by Janis Roszler and Donna Rice. American Diabetes Association; Alexandria, VA, 2007.

WEBSITES

American College of Obstetricians
   and Gynecologists . . . . WWW.ACOG.ORG
   Website of the American College of Obstetricians and Gynecologists.

American Urological Association . . . WWW.AUANET.ORG
   Website of the American Urological Association.

National Diabetes Information
   Clearinghouse . . . . WWW.DIABETES.NIDDK.NIH.GOV/DM/A–Z.ASP
   This section of the National Diabetes Information Clearinghouse website provides an A-to-Z list of diabetes topics.

PUBLICATIONS

National Institutes of Health; *Sexual and Urologic Problems of Diabetes,* NIH Publication 04:5135

CHAPTER 9

DEAL WITH SOME UNEXPECTED PROBLEMS

41. What to expect as a hospitalized patient

42. How to make injections more comfortable and successful

43. How to dispose of sharp things

44. What to throw in the suitcase and the carry-on bag

45. How to prepare for a disaster

What to expect as a hospitalized patient

Illness, infection, pain, and stress typically increase blood glucose levels in patients with type 1 or type 2 diabetes. The numbers can jump quite high in type 1 diabetes, which is why knowing the sick-day rules is important (see Thing to Know 33). If you are admitted to a hospital, expect that your "numbers" may be higher in the hospital than at home. In addition, you will not be on your normal routine (food, activity, etc.), so you may experience some bouncing with your numbers. Tight control may be difficult if you aren't eating well, if you're having tests and procedures that may limit what you can eat, and if you are on bed rest. Your target goal for blood glucose may be adjusted temporarily during your stay. Here are some recommendations and tips about experiencing a hospital stay when you have diabetes:

PREPARING TO BE HOSPITALIZED

BEFORE ADMISSION

1. Write down your current list of medications (diabetes-related, non–diabetes-related, vitamins/minerals, herbal remedies, and over-the-counter medications you take on a daily basis). Write down the exact name, dosage, frequency of dosing, purpose of the drug, and prescribing doctor's name.

➤ Example: "Glucophage, 500 mg, twice a day, morning and night, diabetes medication, Dr. Clark"

2. Record, in brief, any medical conditions for which you have been treated or are currently being treated, with the date(s) and location(s). Include past surgeries or any hospital admissions.
➤ Example: "Carpal tunnel syndrome, diagnosed 1989, had surgery in 1990 to repair at Mercy General Hospital in Greenville, OH, by Dr. George Miller"

3. Write down your emergency contact numbers, including someone who lives close by if possible, describing the relationship you have with that person. Make sure you keep this list updated as addresses and cell phone numbers change.
➤ Example: "Alexandra Hill, daughter, cell phone number 321-123-1234, lives in Sharpsburg, WY"

4. Discuss with your spouse and family about generating a living will and/or power of attorney to help direct your care if you cannot speak for yourself. An attorney, hospital admission personnel worker, or social worker can help provide you with information on these documents. Make sure individuals know where these documents are. Make extra copies to take in case you need to be admitted to a hospital. Most hospitals will retain the original at the first visit, but if you make changes, make sure everyone gets an updated copy.

ON ADMISSION

Pack your bag with the following:

✓ One complete change of clothes
✓ Sleeping attire
✓ Slippers that cover the foot and are non-skid
✓ Toothbrush and toothpaste and other personal toiletries
✓ Hairbrush or comb
✓ Reading book or magazines
✓ Eyeglasses/contacts/hearing aids/dentures with storage containers. Label the storage container with your name. A resealable plastic bag can be used in a pinch. Use a permanent marker to write your name and phone number on the bag just in case.
✓ Small notepad or writing paper with pen (few hospitals have pencil sharpeners)

- ✓ Insurance card(s)
- ✓ Primary physician's name, address, and phone number
- ✓ List of medications (see above)
- ✓ List of medical conditions (see above)
- ✓ Contact numbers (see above)
- ✓ Advanced directives (living wills, power of attorney, etc.)

A SPECIAL NOTE FOR PUMPERS

Be sure to bring pump supplies to the hospital, including spare batteries, reservoirs, tubing, prep pads, tape, and dressings. Hospitals are not required to keep all the different brands of supplies and may have a policy about allowing use of the pump in the facility. Be prepared to provide the physician's name who prescribes your pump rates in case the hospital needs assistance. Be prepared to provide certain information such as when you changed your catheter last and your current basal/bolus rates as well as correction factors and target numbers. Some facilities use insulin pens rather than vials, so bring vials of insulin for refilling your pump just in case. You may need to be disconnected from the pump temporarily if the facility has a policy against their use, or if you are have a test or procedure that may damage your pump (such as certain X-rays and CT scans), or if you become mentally (in too much pain or under anesthesia for surgery) or physically unable to care for the pump.

BE READY TO TALK!

ON ADMISSION, EXPECT MANY QUESTIONS

- Do you have an advanced directive (e.g., a living will)?
- Do you have any allergies (include food[s], medications, and environmental)?
- Do you have sensitivity/allergy to latex products (some medical supplies still contain latex, such as gloves, tapes, and dressings)?
- What is your current height and usual weight?
- Have you had any recent weight changes?
- Past and current health conditions and treatments?
- What are your symptoms?

■ When did your symptoms start?

■ How long have your symptoms been going on?

DURING ADMISSION

✓ Most hospitals will use a hospital version of a blood glucose testing device. The frequency of the testing is determined by your physician responsible for your care. Speak up if you have specific needs regarding frequency or time of day to test. Most likely, the staff will check it two to four times a day. This may be more frequent if you have procedures performed or have a serious illness to treat.

✓ Inform your health care team at the hospital (from the nursing assistant who makes your bed to the doctors) about your unique symptoms of hypoglycemia. Notify them if you suffer from hypoglycemia unawareness (inability to detect when your blood glucose is dropping or low). Typically, hypoglycemia treatment in the hospital is 4 oz of a liquid carbohydrate food (juice, regular soda). You may or may not require a follow-up snack, depending on the severity of your hypoglycemia, the timing of your next meal, your activity, and your medical condition. Inform the staff if you have specific or preferred methods for treating hypoglycemia.

✓ Prepare to have your diabetes medications altered if necessary, based on your condition in the hospital. Know that it is not unusual to be put on insulin short term, even if you were just "diet controlled" or "on pills" at home. Insulin is a preferred medication to treat your diabetes in the hospital because it is quick-acting and can be readily adjusted.

✓ Unlike home, the hospital has dozens or hundreds of people to feed, all at about the same time. Mealtimes may not be what you are used to at home. Be patient with the dietary staff, but certainly inform the staff if you feel any symptoms of hypoglycemia while waiting for your meal tray, or any time you have symptoms.

✓ Because the diet is considered a prescription in the hospital, ask first "what" and "when" it is acceptable to have outside food brought in by well-intentioned family and visitors. Ask to see the registered dietitian on staff if you have special requests or needs (no pork, no tomato products, etc.).

GETTING READY TO GO HOME

ASK A LOT OF QUESTIONS

▮ How often should I check my blood glucose once I am home?

▮ What activities am I allowed to perform? From what activities should I refrain?

▮ What changes (if any) have been made to my home diabetes medications?

▮ What changes (if any) have been made to my other home medications?

▮ Do I have any new prescriptions (ask to be instructed on each drug)?

▮ Who should I call if I have diabetes-related questions after I leave?

▮ What is my plan for follow-up care (next appointments/referrals, etc.)?

▮ What are signs of problems/trouble I should know that would require me to alert my physician?

MORE RESOURCES TO EXPLORE

WEBSITES

AARP . . . . .WWW.AARP.ORG
Website for AARP (formerly know as the American Association of Retired Persons). The section Talking About Your Final Wishes contains information on health decisions and end-of-life choices.

American Hospital Association. . . . . .WWW.AHA.ORG
Website for the American Hospital Association, where you can find "Patient Care Partnership," a brochure on patient rights.

National Instititutes of Health . . . . WWW.NLM.NIH.GOV/MEDLINEPLUS/
ADVANCEDIRECTIVES.HTML
This section of the website of the National Institutes of Health includes directives and informational pamphlet on living wills.

How to make injections more comfortable and successful

Hit the bull's eye. Know what body area is the recommended area to be used for the injection so that it will be used by the body properly. For instance, insulin is to be injected into the fatty layer of tissue (subcutaneous tissue) just under the skin. Injecting insulin into muscle tissue can cause more discomfort, and there will be different absorption of the medication, which can affect your level of control. If you are on any injectable diabetes medication, find out where the best target is for you.

Avoid possible problem areas. Injecting into skin where there is a natural body fold or perspiration may cause irritation. Injecting into skin that has scar tissue or stretch marks may be more difficult and is not recommended because the desired "soft" tissue target may have been replaced by "tough" scar tissue. Avoid hairy body areas, since you may not be able to see as well to begin with, and if an irritation develops, you may not be able to spot it quickly.

It's not cool to be too cool. Allow the medication you are injecting to warm to room temperature. Medications straight out of the refrigerator may sting a bit. At least hold the vial or pen containing the medication in your hand to warm it up for a minute or two.

Keep clean and dry. Cleanse the area with alcohol but allow it to completely dry. Injecting while the alcohol is still wet may cause stinging, since alcohol may get injected along with your insulin. Even tiny amounts can cause irritation.

Pinch up an inch. Find a site where you can pull up about 1 inch or more thickness of fatty tissue. Less than 1 inch indicates the depth of the fatty layer may not be sufficient to receive the needle comfortably, since it may go through a thin layer of fat into more sensitive tissue. You can go too deep.

Size matters. Choose a syringe with the recommended needle size. Thin individuals and children may benefit from thin, short needles. However, these may not be appropriate for everyone. You can also go too shallow, the opposite of what is described above in "pinch up an inch." Some individuals who are overweight, or who have thick skin, may experience absorption problems (as evidenced by poor blood glucose control or injection problems) if they use syringes with short needles. Check with your pharmacist or diabetes educator about the choices that are available.

Avoid leaks. Inject the medication without the medication actively dripping from the needle. Leakage means you are losing medication, and the fluid may cause stinging or localized skin irritation during or after the injection. If your injection device requires you to aspirate (expel a small amount from the needle tip to assure proper measure and flow), gently flick the extra fluid off the tip before attempting the injection.

Darts anyone? Inject at a 90-degree angle (straight in), just like throwing a dart, if normal weight or above normal weight. Use a 45-degree angle (sideways) if you are very thin.

Use fluid movement, not force. Do not use a "heavy hand" to pierce the skin when pushing the needle in or pushing the plunger forward. Use a steady hand to insert the needle and push the plunger smoothly. If you are dispensing a lot of insulin, or go too fast, or are in a not-so-good area (scar tissue area), the insulin may partially seep back out once the needle is withdrawn. It is impossible to know how much insulin you have received; therefore, do not attempt a second injection. Monitor your blood glucose levels frequently and make adjustments in your treatment plan as advised by your health care professional. Avoid that site in the future.

Finish up the right way. Do not aggressively rub or apply pressure just after the injection at the puncture site. It is not necessary to reapply alcohol. Wipe any drop of blood away with a cotton ball. Notify your physician if you have frequent bleeding or more than just a drop.

Use proper needle care. Use a new syringe/pen needle each time for maximum comfort. Syringe needles can be polished or coated with a lubricant to make the injection go smoothly. Once used, the initial "finish" on the syringe has changed and may not be as comfortable. In addition, the needle may be slightly bent, which could affect the angle the next time. The more tissue it passes through, the more possibility of discomfort.

Mark the date and rotate. Rotate injection sites each time, staying at least two fingers width away from the previous site. Lefties tend to abuse the right side of their body target areas out of convenience, and righties tend to abuse the left side. Use a calendar or other tracking system to help you stay in a rotation.

- Discuss any pain, bruising, or bleeding issues with your health care professional if they recur. Avoid the area to prevent further discomfort.
- Report any area that turns red, has a raised surface, has a rash-like appearance, or is tender/sensitive. Some individuals may have sensitivities to components in the medication or the delivery device (allergies or sensitivities).
- Do you have an infection? Notify a health care provider at once if you have an injection site that feels hot, is filled with fluid, or develops into a blister. You may have developed an infection that needs immediate treatment. Some common causes of injection infections are as follows:
  - Reusing the same syringe many times
  - Poor hygiene
  - Using a syringe that has become contaminated (laid on a bathroom surface with the needle exposed)

MORE RESOURCES TO EXPLORE

WEBSITES

The following is a list of companies who manufacture insulin. Information about insulin and how to administer it can be found on these sites:

Sanofi Aventis Pharmaceuticals . . . . WWW.GOINSULIN.COM

Eli Lilly Co. Pharmaceuticals. . . . . WWW.LILLYDIABETES.COM

Novo Nordisk Pharmaceuticals . . . . WWW.CHANGINGDIABETES-US.COM

43

How to dispose of sharp things

KEEP THE EARTH CLEAN

Several groups concerned about public health and the environment are working with officials from local and state governments as well as the Environmental Protection Agency (EPA) to help develop safe strategies for the disposal of home medical waste, including sharps (needles, lancets, syringes, etc.). Sharps pose a public health hazard to workers throughout the waste disposal process, from those who pick up your cans on the curb to those working at the landfill. Syringes have also been found to wash up on the shores of local streams, lakes, and other bodies of water, through improper handling and disposal. This type of polluted waste puts animals at risk as well. Disposing of sharps outside the home also endangers a whole new set of individuals, namely the cleaning and maintenance staff of the building. Punctures, serious wounds, infections, and deadly diseases (hepatitis and HIV, among others) can result from improper contact with used medical sharps. No one wants to be responsible for causing harm from one of his or her own used sharps. Here is information and resources to help you dispose of sharp things more safely.

WHAT ARE THE REGULATIONS?

Check with your local waste management facility to see if they have special requirements or arrangements to dispose of your sharps. Find out from officials in your local and state government if there are guidelines you need to follow. Regulations not only vary from state to state, they can vary among local jurisdictions. Your friend one town over may have different regulations than you do, so be sure to check for your area. No matter what state you live in, open lancets, needles, and syringes (used or unused) should *never* be thrown loose into a regular trash receptacle or flushed into a septic or sewer system. To be a good citizen, choose an option that provides safe containment.

WHAT ARE MY OPTIONS?

- Use designated local used sharp drop-off sites or centers.
- Sign up for special waste removal services through a local waste management company.
- Use a home container mail-back service.
- Use an approved needle destruction device, engineered just for syringe disposal (do not try to make your own, such as bending with pliers or trying to cut your own; injuries may result to you and waste management personnel).
- Contain the sharps.

WHAT DO I DO UNTIL I GET A REGULATION SHARPS CONTAINER?

- Dispose of sharps in a strong plastic or metal container that has a lid that can be securely fastened when full.
- Choose the right size container. If the sharps do not fit easily, spills could occur and closing the container could be difficult.
- Do not use glass (it will shatter and no longer be a container).
- Do not use identifiable recyclable plastic containers, which could be misdirected to a recycling center and pose a hazard.
- Label the container as "MEDICAL WASTE."
- Keep the container out of reach of children and pets.
- Purchase a "home sharps container" available from pharmacies, home medical equipment stores, or specialty diabetes supply mail-order companies.
- Purchase an approved needle destruction device such as BD-Safe Clip, which not only clips, but also contains the used

needle in a nifty receptacle (1-888-BDCARES).

I Consult with your local pharmacist about other options and products.

I Look into resources, such as the BD website at www.bddiabetes.com, which has a listing of state regulations. The EPA has a handout (document EPA 530-F-014) at www.epa.gov/osw titled "Safe Options for Home Needle Disposals."

COMPANIES THAT HAVE MAIL-BACK CONTAINER EXCHANGE PROGRAMS

I Kendall Mail-Away Program (1-800-962-9888)

I BD Sharps Disposal by Mail (1-888-232-2737)

I Sharps Solutions, Sharps Compliance Corporation (1-800-772-5657)

I Medasend Mailback, Inc. (1-800-200-3581)

I GRP Mailback Sharps Disposal (1-800-207-0976)

Others may be available as well. Ask your diabetes educator or pharmacist for further recommendations.

WHAT IF I AM ON THE GO?

I Check into small syringe carrying cases or diabetes supply travel bags designed with straps, or pockets or pouches designed for syringes and supplies.

I Purchase a portable sharps container such as Sharps Transport Tube, from Sharps Compliance (1-800-772-7657).

I Use an empty travel toothbrush holder or a reading glasses–size empty eyeglass case in a pinch.

I Ask your worksite environmental services leader if there is an approved disposal box or station. Chances are, if they don't already have one they will want to make the investment to avoid injury to others.

I Most airports and many government-building restrooms have sharps disposal containers mounted inside. Large private buildings may also—ask.

I An empty vitamin bottle can serve as a small receptacle for used lancets and fit easily in a backpack, briefcase, or purse.

44

What to throw in the suitcase and the carry-on bag

Traveling with diabetes does require some extra planning, but it's not too much trouble. Are you ready for your well-deserved vacation? First of all, to avoid getting a migraine headache at the "check baggage" counter, take time to learn the rules. Check in advance with your transportation carrier (whether it is a plane, train, bus, or shuttle car) about the luggage regulations. Know the legal guidelines as well as find out how your bags will be stored and to what temperatures they will be exposed. Legal guidelines are not the only consideration. Some airlines have their own specific guidelines, so take the time to find out what the current guidelines are. If you are uncertain where to begin, invest in a travel agent to help you.

There are special storage issues for certain diabetes supplies that need to be addressed. The underbelly of the bus or train, or the baggage hold of the plane, may experience extremes in temperatures during travel. Most oral medications and diabetes meters/testing strips are to be stored at room temperature. Some injectables must be kept cool. There are travel bags made specifically for diabetes supplies you can find in the back of diabetes-related magazines or websites. And most have optional cool packs that keep things cooler for hours. You can also create your own using a medium-size cosmetic bag or a shaving kit. Even if you plan putting these things in your carry-on bag, make sure you put your identification on *everything*.

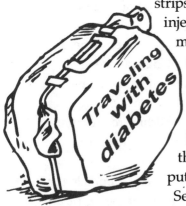

Second, if you are planning a long trip, or one to

a far-off place, have your health care provider write a letter on your behalf, detailing your diabetes care and supply needs. Keep this letter with you at all times. It may also be helpful to get some extra prescriptions, just in case.

Third, as you pack, you will realize you have a bit more "stuff" to squeeze into that bag than before you had diabetes. The key is to have a plan, but be smart, too. Think through what you put in the suitcase and what you will carry with you, since these supplies may be needed right away, or may have to be your sole supply if your luggage doesn't make it. As a general rule, keep your diabetes supplies with you in a carry-on bag—you never know when you might need something. Take more than you usually need. That will give you peace of mind, since you may not have the same ease of access to pharmacies or stores as you do at home. And, unfortunately, if you travel at all, you know there is a risk of damaged, destroyed, and lost luggage once it leaves your sight. If you put all your diabetes gear in the suitcase on your way to Jamaica and it gets sent to Japan instead, you are going to have a not-so wonderful experience in the tropical paradise as you planned. As stated previously, make sure you put your identification on everything. It might be a good idea for you to even write down the brand, size, and color and any unique features (brass tags, designer logos, wheels, etc.) of your luggage on a piece of notepaper in case you have to go to the dreaded "missing luggage" line. They will probably give you a blank or glazed expression if the only description you have of your own luggage is that it is a "black garment bag."

Finally, travel can also upset your normal routine for meals and activity, as well as turn up your stress level. Extra or heavy meals, sitting for long times on a bus, and travel jitters can all raise your blood glucose. Having some snacks of your own can help you prevent overeating or help you fill up when there are delays. Get up and walk or do some movements in your seat to keep your circulation going whenever possible. Stay calm and ask for help when you need it, rather than stressing out if you are having concerns or unmet needs. Cell phones are great when you need a friend. Just pick up the phone and feel connected again if you need a familiar voice to talk over a situation or problem. But don't forget to take your cell phone charger!

WHAT TO LEAVE AT HOME

- ✓ Flip-flops (they are not safe, not stable, and not protective)
- ✓ Visors (don't forget the scalp can burn, too!)
- ✓ Cosmetics/toiletries you have never tried before but bought because they were in a cute little travel size—the last thing you need on vacation is an allergic rash
- ✓ Perishable snacks—they usually get thrown away immediately
- ✓ Snacks that melt (for example, chocolate-covered granola bars)
- ✓ Crumbly snacks (for example, crackers, cookies, and chips) that are packaged wrong (not unless you have a use for crumbs when you get there)
- ✓ Carbonated drinks—the fizz may go crazy after bouncing around in your bag
- ✓ Attitude—wait your turn, be nice to others, and follow your kindergarten rules when you are in the crush trying to get to your final destination

MORE RESOURCES TO EXPLORE

WEBSITES

Amtrak . . . . WWW.AMTRAK.COM
Website for Amtrak rail service.

Greyhound Bus Line . . . . WWW.GREYHOUND.COM
Website for the Greyhound Bus Line.

Federal Aviation Administration . . . . WWW.FAA.GOV
Website for the Federal Aviation Administration, U.S. Department of Transportation, where you can find information on federal airline luggage/ carry-on guidelines.

Transportation Security Administration . . . . . WWW.TSA.GOV
Website of the Transportation Security Administration, U.S. Department of Homeland Security. Especially helpful is the section What To Know Before You Go.

WHAT TO PACK: SUITCASE VERSUS THE CARRY-ON

For the suitcase	For the carry-on
▪ First aid kit containing antibiotic cream, bandages of different sizes, alcohol pads, pain reliever/fever reducer, stomach/ digestive remedies, motion sickness treatments (if needed), cortisone cream, insect repellent, sunburn treatment	▪ Regular and medical ID, insurance cards
	▪ Medications in original containers with your name, medication name, and prescribing health care professional's name in re-sealable plastic bags
	▪ Meter, strips, lancets, lancet device, individually wrapped alcohol pads or disposable antibacterial wipes
	▪ Plain granola bars, crackers/cereal in a supportive container, dried fruit or nuts, trail mix
▪ Sunscreen and sun protection items (hat, cover-ups)	▪ Hypoglycemia treatments (great ones to travel with include tablets and gels; take extra just in case, along with your favorite follow-up snack)
▪ Comfortable and supportive shoes that have already been broken in	▪ Water, if allowed (drink often, since being exposed to forced air [hot or cold] can contribute to dehydration)
	▪ Medical contact information (doctor and pharmacy)
▪ Extra snacks, shelf-stable and temperature-stable, both for the way there and back	▪ Pump supplies (if needed, carry several catheters [and necessary supplies] in case one malfunctions or gets dropped in the dirty airport bathroom floor during insertion)
	▪ Antibacterial disposable wipes (in case you cannot get access to water) or carry a few sets of disposable gloves
▪ Extra syringes and lancets and pump supplies (if you are on the pump, you should still bring syringes, just in case your pump malfunctions)	▪ A portable sharps container (see Thing You Should Know 43, "How to dispose of sharp things")
	▪ Sugar-free gum (it can help keep your mouth moist as well as refreshed after eating)
	▪ **Patience, patience, patience!** Travel can cause frustrations at times. Don't let the small things ruin your trip.

How to prepare for a disaster

Disaster preparedness has become a hot topic over the last several years, especially after 9/11 and destructive hurricanes. While it is everyone's hope to never have to deal with a massive disaster or security threat, it is important to realize that, at any time in the U.S., someone could be at risk for weather-related emergencies, environmental hazards, or a temporary loss of utilities within the home. People with diabetes are taught from initial diagnosis about the importance of planning for each day. Planning ahead for a possible disaster is a recommendation from our government officials, and our schoolchildren practice various types of drills to learn the basics. You may already have recognized the benefits of having a trusty flashlight in an electricity outage, or having a bottle of drinking water during a water pipe repair, but what else should be considered, especially as far as diabetes is concerned? The following list contains suggestions of items to be stored in your home, preferably in a large, covered plastic (non-rusting) container, labeled as "Disaster Kit":

EMERGENCY SUPPLIES

Just for Diabetes

✓ Up-to-date phone numbers of health care providers

✓ Up-to-date list of medications

✓ Extra prescriptions

✓ Backup meter with batteries (charged), strips, lancets (at least a week's supply)

✓ Syringes (if needed, at least a week's supply)

✓ Alcohol pads

✓ Glucagon kit (if recommended by physician)

✓ Hypoglycemia treatments (gels, tablets, or honey; check expiration dates frequently)

✓ Reusable cool packs (keep them in the freezer so you can "grab and go")

✓ Plastic box with tight lid for storing medications if needed

✓ Regular and diet sodas

Just for Basic Needs

✓ Flashlight with extra batteries

✓ Candles, matches, lighters

✓ Disposable gloves

✓ First aid kit

✓ Sterno cans

✓ Water (1 gallon/day/person)

✓ Sanitizing gels

✓ Disposable baby wipes

✓ Battery-operated radio with extra batteries

✓ Emergency battery-operated cell phone charger

✓ Shelf-stable food stuffs

✓ Paper towels/toilet paper

✓ Disposable utensils

✓ Can opener

✓ Utility knife (with attachments)

✓ Blankets

✓ Extra clothing

TIPS FOR PREPARING FOR A DISASTER

▌Stay informed during threatening weather conditions or events by listening to the radio or television.

▌Make and discuss a disaster plan with household members and family members on a calm day.

▌Discuss escape routes from the home and evacuation road routes with household members in advance. Try some drills to see how your plan works out. Make sure everyone knows where your supply kit is.

▌Get training in first aid and CPR from your local Red

Cross chapter or health care facility.

∎ Don't forget about daily needs of young children (diapers) and other adults (health aids and equipment) and pets (pet food and water).

MORE RESOURCES TO EXPLORE

WEBSITES

American Red Cross. . . . . WWW.REDCROSS.ORG
  Website for the American Red Cross.

Department of Homeland Security. . . . . WWW.READY.GOV
  Website for the U.S. Department of Homeland Security.

CHAPTER 10

AVOID FEELING "LABELED"

How to tell someone you have diabetes

When you get diagnosed with diabetes, it is not uncommon to feel a sense of change regarding your identity. You may have feelings of loss about your "previous" lifestyle, as well as concerns about your current situation and what the future may bring. Diabetes is not who you are, but a health condition that you have. Diabetes is known as a self-management disease, because the person who has the most power to affect the care is the person who *has* diabetes. Therefore, your own attitude will set the stage for how others will react. Here are some ways you can help others around you adjust to your diagnosis in a positive and supportive way.

Remember who you are. You haven't changed. You have a few more things on your to-do list than before, but you are the same person. You may wonder if people will treat you like a sick person if you tell them that you have diabetes. There may be a few nitwits around who have their own personal hang-ups or issues that cannot be changed, but you will find that those who truly care about you will continue to care about you just like before. Show them you can stay healthy by following your medical management plan and fight the "sick" label.

Take your time when telling others about your diabetes. You may need to take time to make the adjustment yourself before including others.

Give people a chance to be supportive. You may worry that others around you may badger you if you dare to eat a cookie, or harass you in a less than supportive way to exercise if you tell them you have diabetes. Think about the role you need to play in your care and how others can help you. Communicate these wishes to them up front so they know what they can do to help you, rather than let the "food police" or the "exercise taskmaster" come out of nowhere.

Show who's in charge. When dealing with a diabetes challenge, small or large, be in command. Tell yourself, "This is what I am going to do to solve this problem," rather than, "Poor me, there is nothing I can do myself."

Beware of the joker. There is always more than one jokester out there who will undoubtedly fire comments out such as, "Well, I guess you can't eat those candy bars anymore, can you? Just give them to me! Ha, ha!" or, "You won't be coming to happy hour with us anymore, will you?" Recognize that some people have a poor sense of humor at times, and shrug it off. Comments like that can't hurt you if you don't take the joker seriously.

Talk to someone who knows. Talk to someone who has diabetes already if you want an empathetic ear. Join a support group, or log on to a blog site to fight the feelings of isolation that sometimes occur with a diagnosis of diabetes.

Educate others. Some individuals have considerable anxiety about "having a low" in front of their friends or coworkers. They believe if it were to occur, it would be an embarrassment and create a stigma. If you educate those who are closest to you personally and on the job, you will find most people are eager to help if they know how.

The relationship may change for the better. Telling a friend about your diabetes will build a new aspect to your relationship. It will help to develop support and understanding between the two of you.

Not everyone needs to know. It is important to tell all the members of your health care team—the pharmacist, dentist, optometrist/oph-thalmologist, OB/GYN, etc., so they can provide you with the appropriate level of care for your health needs. It would also be beneficial to tell family members about diabetes, since it does tend to run in families, and others may benefit from knowing their risk for preventative action or for possible screening themselves. But, there are some people in your life who do not need ever know, and you have the right not to share your personal health information with them.

Express your feelings. Let people know how you feel about having diabetes so they can better understand where you are coming from.

47

How to have a night out with friends

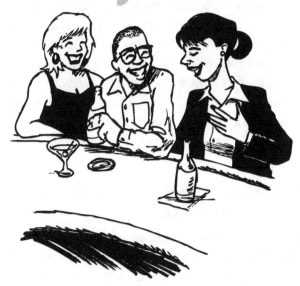

If you like to have a drink at family gatherings, parties, or after work at the local club, you need to understand how alcohol affects your body and your blood glucose when you have diabetes. First of all, ask your physician whether or not alcohol is acceptable for your current health status. Despite the current research stating one to two drinks a day may help reduce your risk of heart disease, daily alcohol is not appropriate for some health conditions. Alcohol may worsen problems with high blood pressure (hypertension), some forms of diabetic neuropathy, and high triglycerides (hypertriglyceridemia). Alcohol can also affect how medications work; therefore, *ask first* to stay out of danger. Interactions with some medications and alcohol can be very serious.

WHY SHOULD I BE CONCERNED ABOUT ALCOHOL?

Diabetes is a disease where your metabolism is not working properly. Alcohol can also affect the metabolism, so you are at additional risk of having a metabolic imbalance if you drink alcohol. Here's a brief review of how alcohol affects the body:

Alcohol does not use the normal digestive process to be metabolized (used) in the body. Unlike food, which needs the stomach and intestines to break it down into pieces of fuel to then enter the bloodstream for energy, alcohol enters your bloodstream within minutes of being ingested. The liver then takes responsibility for breaking down the alcohol and will prioritize taking care of the alcohol above its normal duties. The liver has an important role in maintaining glucose levels in the blood. The liver can help release glucose back into the bloodstream when needed, to help prevent or correct a dropping blood glucose level. When alcohol is present, it sets aside this task and tries to process the alcohol first. Because of this, alcohol can increase your risk of having a low blood glucose reaction, or a more severe reaction if your blood glucose is already dropping.

SOME SUGGESTIONS ABOUT DRINKING ALCOHOL WHEN YOU HAVE DIABETES

■ Eat something with your alcoholic beverage. By providing some food energy with the alcohol, hopefully the two will balance each other out and help prevent a low blood glucose. Have your wine at mealtime; or if you have a cocktail, have an appetizer to go along with it.

■ If you like mixed drinks, choose mixers that are calorie free, such as diet sodas, diet tonic, or seltzer waters. Make sure you impress upon the bartender this is your request. Take a small sip at first to make sure they mixed it right.

■ Keep a low blood glucose treatment kit (source of carbohydrate) on you if you are drinking away from home.

■ Do not drink if you plan to become pregnant or you are pregnant.

- Check your blood glucose before going to bed after consuming alcohol. Alcohol can affect your blood glucose many hours later, so keep a low blood glucose treatment just beside the bed, just in case you wake feeling low.
- Do not perform vigorous physical activity while drinking alcohol. This combination will significantly increase your risk of having hypoglycemia, since activity also lowers blood glucose levels.

NUTRITION CONTENT OF VARIOUS DRINKS

Below is a chart with some estimates of nutrition contents of certain alcoholic beverages. In the future, we may see nutrition labeling on all alcoholic beverages. The laws on labeling at least state that "light" or "lite" beverages must provide information about carbohydrate or calories. "Low-carb" beverages must contain no more than 7 grams per serving.

Drink	Serving	Calories	Carbo-hydrate	Protein	Calories from Alcohol
Table wine, 11.5% alcohol	5 oz	124	4 g	0 g	108
Champagne	4 oz	78	1 g	0 g	72
Red wine	5 oz	129	5 g	0 g	107
White wine	4 oz	113	7 g	0 g	86
Dessert wine, sweet	3.5 oz	165	14 g	0 g	110
Sherry	1 oz	45	3 g	0 g	32
Light wine, 6% alcohol	5 oz	74	2 g	0 g	66
Liquors, whiskey, scotch, distilled, 90 proof, 45% alcohol	1 oz	73	0 g	0 g	73
Liquor, vodka, distilled, 80 proof, 40% alcohol	1.5 oz	97	0 g	0 g	97
Beer	12 oz	153	13 g	2 g	98
Light beer	12 oz	103	6 g	0 g	77
Nonalcoholic beer	12 oz	65	13 g	0 g	7

Source: Calorie King, www.calorieking.com, accessed May 2008.

■ Stop at two drinks if you're a man, one if you're a woman. Sip them slowly to make them last. Standard drink sizes are as follows: beer, 12 oz; wine, 5 oz; and liquor/80 proof or higher, 1 1/2 oz.

CHOOSING NOT TO DRINK, BUT STILL FEELING LIKE PART OF THE CROWD

Ask for "virgin" drinks at the bar, or have the bartender add some fruit garnishes to club soda or your diet soft drink to liven it up. Snack on appetizers lightly unless you plan to modify your meal plan. Some lower-fat choices are pretzels, baked chips, vegetables, and grilled meats or seafood. If you plan to dance or bowl, or have other physical activity, and it has been a while since your meal, snack on an appetizer to help keep you fueled and your blood glucose in balance. Use your sparkling personality, not alcohol, to help feel part of the crowd.

HELP FOR PROBLEMS WITH ALCOHOL

If you feel you are consuming more alcohol than you should, or feel you are becoming dependent on alcohol to feel happy or relaxed on a regular basis, seek help. Inform your health care professional. Help is available. The sooner you can get assistance, the better. If you feel like you have a problem, you probably do. Here are some additional resources:

■ Alcoholics Anonymous, 1-212-870-3400, www.alcoholics-anonymous.org. Check your phone book for a local chapter.
■ National Institute on Alcohol Abuse and Alcoholism, 1-301-443-3860, www.niaaa.nih.gov.
■ National Drug and Alcohol Treatment Referral Routing Service (Federal Substance Abuse Program), 1-800-662-HELP.

MORE RESOURCES TO EXPLORE

MAGAZINES, JOURNALS, AND OTHER PERIODICALS

"Alcohol and the Low-Carb Myth," University of California–
Berkeley Wellness Letter, August 2004,
http://www.wellnessletter.com/html/wl/2004/wlFeature0804.html.

BOOKS

Harmful Interactions: Mixing Alcohol with Medicines. NIH Publication No.
03-5329, revised 2007.

WEBSITES

American Diabetes Association . . . . WWW.DIABETES.ORG
   *The website for the American Diabetes Association contains a wealth of
   nutrition information, including sections on alcohol and diabetes.*

dLife . . . . WWW.DLIFE.COM
   The website for dLife. Be sure to check out the section Diabetes and Alcohol.

48

How to recognize the blues

WHAT ARE THE BLUES?

From time to time in everyone's life, there are experiences that can lead us to feeling down and out. Sometimes the days seem rather dark and dismal. Thankfully, these occasions are few and far between for most people. It is normal to have some negative feelings from time to time, whether you have diabetes or not—stuff happens. These feelings usually pass after a few days, and you feel better.

WHAT IS DEPRESSION?

Depression is a disorder when negative feelings and mood start to influence or interfere with issues in your daily life, such as eating, sleeping, work, and relationships. Sometimes depression is short-lived and occurs after a negative experience or unexpected tragedy or loss. But at other times, the problems do not resolve, or gets worse.

WHAT ARE SOME SYMPTOMS OF DEPRESSION?

- Feeling tired all the time
- Sleep disorders (sleeping more or less than usual)
- Eating/appetite changes (eating more or less than usual)

- Feelings of sadness, helplessness, or loss
- Negative feelings about yourself or your future
- Difficulty in remembering things or concentrating
- Moodiness
- Social changes (wanting to be alone or fears about being alone)

DOES HAVING DIABETES MAKE IT MORE LIKELY I WILL GET DEPRESSION?

Yes, research has shown that individuals with a chronic disease such as diabetes are more likely to have depression. There are several reasons why this may occur:

1. The individual may be having a bad reaction to the diagnosis. Individuals experience a variety of feelings after learning about a new health condition. When the diagnosis is diabetes, a chronic lifelong disease, the news can hit hard. Some individuals may feel mad, others may be tearful, and others may be relieved that the diagnosis is not any worse than diabetes, if they have been feeling bad for some time. Emotional imbalance may contribute to internal stress.

2. Individuals with diabetes pay a lot more "attention" to their daily activities, which can seem cumbersome at times.

3. Individuals with diabetes may experience more challenges with maintaining good health overall and possibly face secondary problems such as hypertension, heart disease, kidney disease, and others.

4. Chronic diseases require ongoing medical care, which may cause a disruption in one's daily schedule as well as affect financial status.

5. Blood glucose changes can affect a person's mood, feelings, and energy level, especially if blood glucose levels are not well controlled. This fuel imbalance may cause some minor negative feelings to worsen by contributing to moodiness and fatigue.

WILL MY DOCTOR THINK I AM CRAZY
IF I THINK I HAVE DEPRESSION?

No. Depression is a common disorder and must be treated as any other health condition. If you do not have a strong relationship with your doctor, but feel comfortable with talking with the nurse or medical assistant in the office, express your concerns to them and let them know you want their help in opening the doors to communication. Your medical record is private, and no one will have access to it unless you grant it.

WILL MY FRIENDS AND FAMILY THINK I AM WEAK
IF I NEED HELP FOR DEPRESSION?

Contrary to past myths, true depression is not something you can just "snap out of." It will take time. Ignore the myths and any "quick-fix" advice you might be given, such as "just take a day off, and you'll feel better." Seek out professional medical care for advice and treatment.

WHAT ARE TREATMENTS FOR DEPRESSION?

- *Counseling*. Counseling should be performed by a licensed professional specializing in psychology or psychiatry. The sessions may be covered under your health care plan, or reduced-cost or free services may be available to you if you are eligible for certain programs. Some employers offer Employee Assistance Programs with health care services as a free or low-cost benefit to employees. Ask about coverage.
- *Medications*. There are a wide variety of medications that are available to treat depression. Avoid trying to use caffeine or herbal products as a self-prescribed treatment, since they may cause you more harm than good. Some herbal products are dangerous to take with prescription medications, so follow advice about medications from a licensed health care professional only.
- *Education*. Depression can reoccur. It is important for you to learn how to recognize your own symptoms of depression, so that if they begin, you can seek assistance early on and hopefully recover sooner. Develop a plan to help prevent relapses, and use that plan when symptoms start.

RESOURCES FOR DEPRESSION AND TREATMENT OPTIONS

▮ Licensed psychologists

▮ Licensed psychiatrists

▮ Licensed mental health counselors

▮ Mental health programs (city or state)

▮ Support groups

▮ Employee assistance programs

▮ Social services

MORE RESOURCES TO EXPLORE

MAGAZINES, JOURNALS, AND OTHER PERIODICALS

"10 Steps for Coping With a Chronic Condition." 2003. Harvard Heart Letter, Harvard Health Publications, Harvard Medical School, http://www.health.harvard.edu/heart, accessed May 2008.

Coping with Chronic Illness. Patient Information Publication, 1996. Warren Grant Magnuson Clinical Center, National Institutes of Health; Bethesda, MD.

Dealing with Diabetes Diagnosis as an Older Adult. 2004. National Diabetes Education Program, U.S. Department of Health and Human Services, National Institutes of Health, and Centers for Disease Control. Found at www.ndep.nih.gov or ordered by contacting NDEP.

BOOKS

Chicken Soup for the Soul, Healthy Living Series: Diabetes, by Jack Canfield, Mark Hansen, and Bryon Hoogwerf. HCI Publications. The Cleveland Clinic; Cleveland, OH, 2006.

WEBSITES

Cleveland Clinic Foundation . . . . WWW.CLEVELANDCLINIC.ORG
Website for the Cleveland Clinic Foundation, Health Information Center. The section Chronic Illness and Depression is especially helpful.

National Institutes of Mental Health. . . . . WWW.NIMH.NIH.GOV
Website for the National Institutes of Mental Health.

How to keep a positive attitude

Some people seem to always be smiling, even on rainy days. Perhaps it is their unique natural personality, or it is a daily decision to be on the sunny side of life. Here are some tips to help reach and sustain a positive attitude when living with diabetes.

Stay active. Research has shown that active people have lower rates of depression and better overall health. Make activity a priority in your life. Exercise causes physiological changes (release of endorphins), which can give you a "power boost" and a feeling of well-being.

Get a hobby. Hobbies are a great way to reduce stress and find personal enjoyment. If you don't already have one, take a walk through a hobby or craft store, or take a class in a subject that has been of interest to you. Can't think of anything? Go with a friend or relative to theirs. You may find you like it, too, or become inspired to branch out on your own.

Smile. Smiling is a great way to show people you are in control. It will likely be returned, which will double the benefits.

Have a stress management plan. There are still going to be "blue Mondays" out there. Have a strategy in advance so that if you hit a speed bump, you won't lose your wheel. A suggestion may be that if you know you might end up having to work overtime on Thursday, try to get a little more rest Wednesday night, or pamper yourself a bit more to be better able to handle the next day.

Forgive and forget. Try to forgive and forget the shortcomings in yourself as well as others. No one is perfect, and no one expects you to have "perfect" blood glucose levels every day. You have to be able to pick yourself up after a situation and move on. Stewing about it will not make today or tomorrow any better. Set your sights on today and move on.

Keep busy. They say many people who retire are often at risk of depression because they have been typically so busy for so long, they feel a sense of boredom once retired. Days can become too routine. If you have those feelings, try to add in some extras into your schedule such as joining a weekly book club, volunteering at a local charity, assisting with a need at your church or local school, adding a small part-time job, or starting a walking club in your own neighborhood.

Get plenty of rest. Sleep recharges a person both mentally and physically. You are better able to fight off stress when you are well rested. Most adults still need about 8 hours of sleep. Staying on a regular bedtime routine will help avoid sleep disorders.

Don't play the numbers. Don't worry about one-time high readings, or a reading that is "off" from your normal. Remember blood glucose readings are data points or information pieces only. It is not a measure of your personality or character. Don't let the numbers cause you to label yourself as "good" or "bad." There may be factors contributing to your numbers that you have little control over, such as having an illness. Use the data—don't *be* the data.

Confide in someone. If you are having some emotional stress, talk to a friend, pastor, family member, or health care professional about your feelings. Sometimes you suddenly feel better after you "talk it out."

Start each day with a positive, or two:

1. Tune your clock radio to a positive or upbeat radio station to wake up to.
2. Read a few lines of poetry before rolling out of bed.
3. Write in a personal journal each day, describing what you think today will bring and how you can make it happen.
4. Read something inspirational or listen to a "book on tape/CD" as you do your morning routine.

5. Spend time with your pet in the morning. By cuddling up or enjoying a walk together, your pet can help reduce your stress levels.

6. Spend a few minutes in quiet reflection or prayer.

7. Read the comics first in the morning newspaper to give yourself a chuckle. You may not want to read anything else!

8. Turn lights on to help your body wake to the new day.

9. Eat breakfast—skipping breakfast may cause you to feel sluggish rather than fueled up. If you can't eat a huge meal, eat a small one to get some nutrition for your body's need for energy.

10. Slip a positive quote or note to yourself, or a small memoir in your briefcase or lunch bag to cheer you midday. Or call your loved ones for a quick hello and tell them you love them. The act of giving always makes a person feel good.

BOOKS TO HELP YOU DEAL WITH EMOTIONAL STRESS

Title	Author	Publisher, Date of Publication
Caring for the Diabetic Soul	Neal Friedman	American Diabetes Association, 1997
101 Tips for Coping with Diabetes	Richard Rubin	American Diabetes Association, 2003
Diabetes Burnout: What To Do When You Can't Take it Anymore	William Polonsky	American Diabetes Association, 1999
Psyching Out Diabetes: A Positive Approach to Your Negative Emotions, 3rd ed.	Richard Rubin, June Biermann, Barbara Toohey	McGraw-Hill Publishing, 1999
Living With Diabetes: Nicole Johnson, Miss America 1999	Nicole Johnson	Lifeline Press, 2001

50

What the future has in store

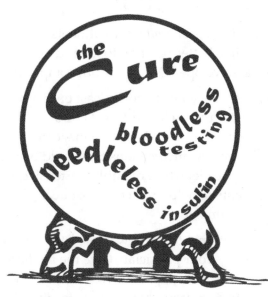

Despite all the knowledge of great scientists who are working on various diabetes research projects all over world, no one knows for sure what diabetes care will look like 5 or 10 years into the future. At best, we can make some educated guesses about future technology and treatments. Naturally, we all hope to someday find a cure, for both type 1 and type 2 diabetes. By current predictions, the world faces an epidemic of new cases of diabetes in the next 10–15 years, given existing rates in both third-world and developed nations.

WHAT DO WE KNOW TODAY?

Currently, activity and research is directed at the following goals:
1. Developing alternative ways to take insulin, such as through a pill or patch rather than by injections
2. Creating "bloodless" glucose meters
3. Exploring pancreatic islet cell transplantation
4. Linking blood glucose meter technology with insulin pumps (closed-loop delivery systems)
5. Preventative medications/treatments for type 1 and type 2 diabetes

WHAT SHOULD I DO TODAY?

✓ *Keep yourself in optimal health.* If treatments do become available, you may be in a better position to take advantage of them if you have not yet developed serious health complications.

✓ *Keep informed.* Ask your doctor at least once a year about what is new in diabetes research and care. Find out if there are any new insights you can use to make self-management easier. Question if there are any new medications that could be used for preventing complications (use of antihypertensive agents or lipid-lowering agents to help protect against heart disease and kidney disease, for example).

✓ *Be flexible.* Be willing to try new advice or a new medication if prescribed by your physician. Give the medications a fair chance—taking them just for a week may not be long enough for the benefits to be measurable. Provide feedback to your doctor if you do not see benefits, or if you have side effects from the medication after a reasonable amount of time. Check with a pharmacist about how long it should take for medications to be effective.

✓ *Two may be better than one; three may be better than two.* There are different types of diabetes medications now available. Some may work with insulin production levels in your pancreas, whereas others may work on your liver (an organ that has key responsibilities in glucose control), or on your gastrointestinal tract (active compounds in your tract can affect your metabolism). Don't flip out if your doctor has you taking several medications—the proof is whether or not your A1C is in the proper level.

✓ *Be a player.* Contribute to your local diabetes charities, which provide funding for research. The government supports hundreds of different health research organizations and cannot put all its monies into only a chosen few. Donations from the public can play a significant part in an organization's research budget.

✓ *Be an advocate.* Stand up for your rights within the health care system and public domain. The American Diabetes Association (ADA) has a dedicated Advocacy division, which can help inform you of current laws and provide useful information to help navigate the often confusing world of politics and policies. Call ADA at 1-888-DIABETES, or visit www.diabetes.org to learn more about advocacy.

✓ *Spread the word.* Encourage others around you to find out if they are at risk for developing diabetes. ADA estimates one-third of people who have diabetes are still undiagnosed. Help with a workplace screening or diabetes information brown-bag lunch lecture. Or, call your local ADA chapter to see how you can help spread the word in your neighborhood, church, and community.

✓ *Live for today.* Find the good in each day, and learn to let the little things go.

> *When one door closes, another door opens; but we so often look so long and so regretfully upon the closed door, that we do not see the ones which open for us.*
>
> **—Alexander Graham Bell**

> *Finish each day and be done with it. You have done what you could; some blunders and absurdities have crept in; forget them as soon as you can. Tomorrow is a new day; you shall begin it serenely and with too high a spirit to be encumbered with your old nonsense.*
>
> **—Ralph Waldo Emerson**

> *It's not what if, it's what now.*
>
> **—Author Unknown**

Index

A

A1C. *See* Hemoglobin A1C test
abscess, 190
acupuncture, 211
aerobic exercise, 89–90
alcohol, 177, 202, 222, 257–260
alternative site testing, 44, 50, 54–56
American Academy of
    Ophthalmology, 216
American Diabetes Association
    (ADA), 6, 81, 271
American Diabetes Association Rec-
    ognized Provider, 7
American Dietetic Association, 21
American with Disabilities Act, 81
amputation, 210
anodyne treatment, 211
aspirin therapy, 222–223

B

back problems, 212
bacteria, 217
bathing, 131–133
batteries, 45–46, 48
bee stings, 198
biofeedback, 212

blister, 197, 211
blood glucose levels. *See also* hyper-
    glycemia; hypoglycemia;
    self-monitoring blood glucose
    (SMBG)
    alcohol, 258–260
    carbohydrates, 103–106
    food, effect on, 111
    Hemoglobin A1C test, 11–17, 146,
        225
    hospitalization, 235
    illness, 187
    infections, 181–182
    ketones, 164
    maintaining good, 184
    menstrual cycle, 158–159
    physical activity, 86
    precautions, 126–131
    pregnancy, 200
    recording, 59–62
    roller coaster readings, 173–177
    sexual health, 229
    at work, 82
blood glucose testing. *See* self-
    monitoring blood glucose
    (SMBG)
blood pressure, 87, 148, 225
blood vessels, 214

bloodstream, 181–182
BMI (body mass index), 225
breakfast, 70, 109
bronchial infection, 190
burns, 196, 211

C

calibration, 43–44, 49
calluses, 211
Calorie Counting, 103
Candida albicans, 183
canker sores, 216
Carbohydrate Counting, 103, 107
carbohydrates, 101–107
cataracts, 214–215
Certified Diabetes Educator (CDE), 7,
    20–21
Charcot foot, 212
cholesterol, 148, 225
circulation, 68, 131, 181–182
cleanliness, 131, 182–183, 208
clothing, 70, 133, 137, 207
coding, 43–44, 49
color vision exam, 215
communication, 126
continuous glucose monitoring
    (CGM), 16
counseling, 264

D

"dawn phenomenon", 69, 76
dental care, 71, 76, 216–218, 224
depression, 262–265
diabetes
    complications, 11
    diagnosis, 255–256, 263
    education, vii–viii, 9
    management, 67–76, 145–148,
        270–271

research, 269
type 1, 69, 161–164
type 2, 69, 161–164
Diabetes Control and Complications
    Trial (DCCT), 11
"diabetic coma". *See* diabetic
    ketoacidosis (DKA)
diabetic ketoacidosis (DKA), 86, 161,
    164–165
diabetic nephropathy, 148, 154
diabetic neuropathy, 130, 132, 139, 154,
    185, 209–213, 218
diabetic retinopathy, 87, 154, 214–215
diarrhea, 189
digestive system, 103
dining out, 78–79, 114–116
disabilities, 81
disaster preparedness, 250–252
discrimination, 80–81
doctor, 3–9, 26–29
doctor of optometry (OD), 215–216
driving, 127

E

education, 264
emergencies, 27–28, 75, 82, 125, 170–
    171, 250–252
emotional health, 266–268, 270–271.
    See also depression
employment, 78–82
endocrinologist, 6, 13, 213
equipment, 4, 32–33, 37–38, 41–52
estimated average glucose (eAG),
    14–15
estrogen, 157
evening routine, 73–76
Exchange/Choice Lists, 103
exercise, 62, 71, 83–93, 169, 204.
    See also physical activity
eye exam, 147, 202, 215
eyes, 154, 198, 214–216

F

Family and Medical Leave Act (FMLA), 81
fast food, 114–115
fat, 101–103
feet, 68, 87, 126, 133–137, 147, 154, 185, 197, 207–208. *See also* diabetic neuropathy
fever, 188
finger-stick testing, 53–55. *See also* self-monitoring blood glucose (SMBG)
first aid, 184
fish, 223–224
fish oil, 223
flexibility exercise, 90
food, 62, 73–74, 97–107, 109–111, 113–116, 192–193, 221
food diary, 23. *See also* logbook
Food Pyramid, 103
fungal infections, 216

G

gait problems, 212
gastroparesis, 69
glaucoma, 214–215
glomerular filtration rate (GFR), 148
glucagon emergency kit, 75
glucose, 161
glucose meters, 37–38, 41–52
glucose testing. *See* self-monitoring blood glucose (SMBG)
Glycemic Index (GI), 104–105
Glycemic Load (GL), 105
goals, 22
gum disease, 71, 76, 216, 224

H

hammertoe, 212
health care team. *See also* main headings e.g. physicians
  alcohol, 260
  blood glucose levels, 62
  Carbohydrate Counting, 107
  choosing a, 5–7
  contacting your, 26–27
  dental care, 218
  depression, 264
  diabetes, 256
  diabetes education, vii–viii
  diabetic neuropathy, 212–213
  exercise, 92
  feet, 138
  foot care, 147
  hospitalization, 238
  infections, 184–185
  meal plan, 110
  medication, 142
  nervous system, 219
  pregnancy, 201–202
  proactive participation, 270–271
  sexual health, 227–229
  vision, 215–216
health insurance. *See* insurance
heart disease, 148, 154, 221–225
heart rate, 87
hemoglobin, 12
Hemoglobin A1C test, 11–17, 146, 225
hobbies, 266
hormones, 157. *See also* insulin
hospitals, 7, 235–239
hyperglycemia
  alternative site testing, 44
  damage from, 130–131
  "dawn phenomenon", 69
  diabetic ketoacidosis (DKA), 165
  driving, 39

R

Recognized Education Program, 21
registered dietitian (RD), 18–25, 98.
    See also Certified Diabetes
    Educator (CDE); health care
    team
resources
    alcohol, 260–261
    blood glucose levels, 17, 178
    Carbohydrate Counting, 107–108
    dental care, 220
    depression, 265
    diabetes management, 63–64,
        71–72, 77, 129, 149
    diabetic neuropathy, 213
    disaster preparedness, 252
    employment, 82
    exercise, 88, 92–93
    foot care, 140, 208
    health care team, 21, 29
    heart disease, 226
    hospitalization, 239
    hypoglycemia, 172
    illness, 190, 194
    infections, 186
    injections, 242
    injuries, 199
    insurance, 34
    ketones, 166
    labor laws, 80–81
    meal plan, 99, 105, 108, 112, 117
    medical care, 9–10
    medication, 144
    menstrual cycle, 160
    physician, choosing a, 6–7
    pregnancy, 204
    registered dietitian (RD), 25
    self-monitoring blood glucose
        (SMBG), 40, 46, 57
    sexual health, 231
    skin care, 134
    smoking cessation program, 156
    travel, 248
    vision, 220
    weight loss, 121
restaurants, 115–116
resting heart rate (RHR), 87
retina, 214
retinal scan, 215
retinopathy. *See* diabetic retinopathy
routines. *See* diabetes, management

S

saliva, 217
self-management, vii–viii
self-monitoring blood glucose
    (SMBG), 16–17, 37–40, 48–57,
    60–62, 76, 79, 173–177. *See also*
    glucose meters
serving sizes, 105, 222
sexual dysfunction, 228–230
sexual health, 227–228
sharps container, 51, 243–245
shoes, 70, 137–138, 185, 207. *See also*
    feet
sinus infection, 190
skin care, 68, 76, 126, 130–133, 199, 208
sleep, 39, 76, 267
slit lamp, 215
smoking. *See* tobacco
smoking cessation program, 155–156
snacks, 73–74. *See also* meal plan
social events, 257
Somogyi effect, 69, 76
sore throat, 188–189
storage, 51
strength exercise, 90
stress, 177, 202, 230, 266–268
stroke, 148

sunburn, 196

supplies. *See also* equipment

    disaster preparedness, 251–252

    illness, 191–193

    morning routine, 71

    pregnancy, 202

    self-monitoring blood glucose (SMBG), 42–46, 49–51

    travel, 247, 249

    urine ketone testing, 162

    at work, 78

support group, 71, 154–155, 255–256. *See also* Certified Diabetes Educator (CDE); health care team; registered dietitian (RD)

syringes, 241–245. *See also* medical waste disposal; sharps container

T

technology, 4, 60

teeth, 71, 76, 148, 154, 197, 216–218

tobacco, 146, 153–156, 207, 230

toe alignment, 212

toothache, 197

travel, 246–249

trends, 60–61

triglycerides, 222, 225

troubleshooting, 52

tuning fork, 147

U

urinary tract infections (UTI), 185

urine ketone testing, 162–166, 203

urologist, 228

V

vaccines, 219

vaginal dryness, 230

vision, 147, 154, 202

vision screening, 215

vitreous, 214

vomiting, 189–190

W

warranties, 42, 48

warts, 198

weight, 118–121, 201, 225

weight loss programs, 119–121

work, 78–82

wounds, 190

Y

yeast infections, 183

OTHER TITLES FROM THE AMERICAN DIABETES ASSOCIATION

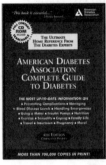

American Diabetes Association Complete Guide to Diabetes, 4th Edition
by American Diabetes Association
Have all the tips and information on diabetes that you need close at hand. The world's largest collection of diabetes self-care tips, techniques, and tricks for solving diabetes-related problems is back in its fourth edition, and it's bigger and better than ever before.
Order no. 4809-04; New low price $19.95

Diabetes 911: How to Handle Everyday Emergencies
by Larry A. Fox, MD, and Sandra L. Weber, MD
When it comes to a condition as serious as diabetes, the best way to solve problems is to prevent them from ever happening. Do you know what to do in case of an emergency? With *Diabetes 911*, you will learn the necessary skills to handle hypoglycemia, insulin pump malfunctions, natural disasters, travel, depression, and sick days.
Order no. 4887-01; Price $12.95

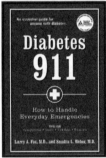

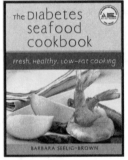

The Diabetes Seafood Cookbook
by Barbara Seelig-Brown
Seafood is the perfect choice for anyone looking to eat healthfully without skimping on flavor. From freshwater and saltwater fish to crab, shrimp, and clams, this book delivers over 150 delicious recipes for the perfect party appetizer, a delightful family dinner, or a satisfying side dish.
Order no. 4670.01; Price $18.95

Ultimate Diabetes Meal Planner
by Jaynie Higgins and David Groetzinger
Fitness and nutrition expert Jaynie Higgins takes the guesswork out of diabetes meal planning and puts every-thing you need in one amazing collection. With 16 weeks of meal plans and over 300 amazing recipes, this book will guide you toward a healthy, diabetes-friendly lifestyle. You'll find meal plans in four different calorie levels and shopping lists to make grocery shopping a breeze. Take the mystery out of food in just 4 easy steps!
Order no. 4725-01; Price $21.95

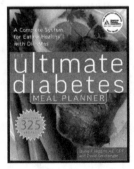

To order these and other great American Diabetes Association titles, call 1-800-232-6733 or visit http://store.diabetes.org.
American Diabetes Association titles are also available in bookstores nationwide.